Indian Medical Science Series No. 52

NATUROPATHY

The Art of Drugless Healing

V.M. Kulkarni

Sri Satguru Publications
a division of
Indian Books Centre
Delhi–India

Published by:
Sri Satguru Publications
Indological and Oriental Publishers
A Division of
Indian Books Centre
40/5, Shakti Nagar,
Delhi-110007
(INDIA)

First Edition : Bombay, 1930
Second Edition : Delhi, 1986, 1997

ISBN 81-7030-036-3

Published by Sunil Gupta, for Sri Satguru Publications, a division of, Indian Books Centre, 40/5, Shakti Nagar, Delhi-110007, India, and printed at D.K. Fine Art Press, Delhi-110052.

PRINTED IN INDIA

CONTENTS

CHAPTER VIII

Pages

CHAPTER IX

CHAPTER X

The book also contains several illustrations on art paper.

PREFACE

Fresh air, Pure water and bright light
Are Nature's gifts which set us right.

With the advance of civilization mankind is getting weaker day by day. Diseases are increasing in number and are becoming more severe in type. New diseases appear and swell the number of those which defy diagnosis and treatment. The average length of life is shrinking. The rate of sickness shows no appreciable improvement. The boasted science of healing is almost daily enriched by researches and discovery of new remedies, but the art of effecting cures is not able to keep pace with it. This is mainly because the medical profession is adopting measures which tend to suppress disease by means of poisonous drugs instead of intelligently using Nature's bounties which not only cure radically but can also prevent disease permanently.

Fresh air, pure water and bright light are Nature's gifts which are an invaluable aid to perfect health.

The poor and the illiterate especially in villages are shutting their doors against these gifts of Nature through sheer ignorance though there is no dearth of these beneficial bounties where they live. The townsmen in their race for wealth neglect their health and do not take sufficient advantage of these bounties.

Drugs and injections cure one disease but beget another more serious than the original one. They often work havoc on the system more than the disease.

Some centuries ago the average duration of human life was a hundred years but now-a-days we find the majority enter an early grave. All know that death is inevitable but only a few believe that good health is natural and a legitimate heritage of man. Nature is a hard-task master. Those who transgress Her laws cannot escape punishment in the form of disease and illness. Good health is the result and reward of implicit obedience to Her laws.

In the following pages the author has attempted to point out the deleterious effects of poisonous drugs and drastic measures upon the human system and to show in the light of accumulated experience how diseases can safely be treated, cured and also prevented with the aid of Nature's bounties.

The Author

Grant Road, Bombay.

December 1930.

NATUROPATHY

THE ART OF DRUGLESS HEALING

CHAPTER I.

Salutation to Nature

प्रणम्य प्रकृतिं प्रेम्णा प्रणीतुं ग्रन्थमारभे ॥
यस्याः प्रभावतः सर्वे प्राणवन्तो हि प्राणिनः ॥ १ ॥
यत्प्रभावाद् दिवा रात्री ऋतवः प्रभवन्ति ते ॥
वसन्तमदनौ चाऽपि स्वकार्यं कुरुतः सदा ॥ २ ॥

Translation:—I begin this book with a loving bow to Nature whose vitality quickens all living beings, whose power brings round day, night and the seasons and keeps the Spring and Cupid (the god of love) always to their appointed task.

संगं हि नरनारीणामपत्योत्पत्तिकारकम् ॥
प्रेरणाद् घटते यस्या वन्दे तां प्रकृतिं शुभाम् ॥ ३ ॥
बालानां पोषणार्थाय दुग्धं स्त्रीणां कुचद्वये ॥
उत्पादयति या देवी रुधिराद् देहसंस्थितात् ॥ ४ ॥
पोषणायैव सर्वेषां फलानि विविधानि च ॥
उत्पादयति नित्यं या पादपेषु लतासु च ॥ ५ ॥

Translation:—To benevolent Nature, who prompts the procreative intercourse of man and woman, who transforms the blood in the female breast into milk for the nourishment of the infants, and who endows trees and creepers with fruits of different kind to feed all living beings, I make my salutation.

या पोषयति धात्रीव रोगान् हरति सर्वदा ॥
सर्वान् रक्षति मातेव पितेव कुरुते हितम् ॥ ६ ॥
नियोजयति सन्मार्गे सन्मित्रमिव या सदा ॥
सा स्वयम्भूर्जगन्माता भूयान्निश्रेयसाय नः ॥ ७ ॥

Translation:—May that self-existent Universal Mother (Nature) who nurses all like a good nurse, cures all diseases always, protects all like a mother and does good like a father and leads all along the path of rectitude like a faithful friend, minister to the happiness of all of us.

---

1 Naturopathy—Its Theory, Principles and Advantages

Naturopathy signifies the treatment of disease with Nature's resources—her free gifts—such as fresh air, pure water, bright sunlight, proper and timely sleep, natural diet, etc.

Primitive races, before the medicinal uses of plants, minerals and poisons came to be discovered were utilising Nature's gifts for the cure of their ailments. Even now a few followers of Nature, some savages and all lower animals are making use of Nature's bounties in getting rid of their diseases. Some experienced medical men have written books on Naturopathic treatment. But in many cases their treatment is not strictly in accordance with the laws of Nature.

"Kulkarni Naturopathy"

The author has in these pages drawn upon his own experience to show how all diseases can be cured and even prevented with Nature's free gifts made use of in accordance with her own laws and without the help of any drugs. Hence this mode of treatment may be styled as **"Kulkarni Naturopathy"**. Some persons may be incredulous as it is taught in the colleges that drugs are very necessary to destory the bacilli which cause disease. But a Naturopath believes that it is the improper diet and the impurities in the blood caused thereby are the cause of a disease with the bacilli peculiar to it, and advocates that the temple of the human soul must be kept scrupulously clean both internally and externally by leading a natural life.

Disease germs cannot thrive in pure blood, they can live and propagate their species only where there are impurities. Hence the best mode of preventing and healing disease is to keep our body clean and blood pure by ridding them of impurities both external and those generated in the body itself. A Naturopath recognizes microbes as a product of disease rather than a cause. "No disease condition", says Dr. Lindlahr "even apparently hopeless can be pronounced incurable unless all the natural methods of treatment have been given a thorough trial. It is no charlatanic boast, but the simple truth, when we affirm that the various natural methods can and do cure so called incurable diseases, such as tuberculosis, cancer, locomotor ataxia, epilepsy, eczema, neurasthenia, insanity and the worst forms of dyspepsia with constipation always providing that the patient possesses sufficient vitality to react to the treatment and that the destruction of vital parts, and organs has not advanced too far. Hence our claim that while there are incurable patients, there are no incurable diseases."

Theory and Principles of Naturopathy

Nature expels morbid matter and impurities from the system, *first* through the rectum whence the waste food products are evacuated; *secondly* through the urinary organs whence certain acids combined with lime, potash, soda, magnesia and other substances taken from the blood are expelled from the system; *thirdly* through the pores of the skin which expel a good deal of waste matter in the form of perspiration, and *fourthly* through the respiratory organs which sustain life by inhaling the air and by exhaling it charged with carbonic acid gas generated in the body.

If these natural functions are not carried on properly, waste morbid matter remains in the body and becomes a fruitful source of disease. For instance we take food not meant by nature for our consumption and it causes constipation, and several other ailments, we swallow a lot of objectionable drugs and chemicals which stupefy our nervous system and cause an excess of crude lime, soda, potash, etc. in the blood which tax the urinary system to a great extent. We wear tight clothes and don't allow our pores to inhale oxygen from the air and to expel waste matter through perspiration. Some persons do not inhale through the nostrils to oxidise their lungs properly but inhale air through the mouth which is a dangerous habit. One must live therefore in accordance with the laws of Nature, try to cure diseases by obeying Nature only, and should not swallow nor introduce into the system any unnecessary poisons.

A Healthy State

A human body is said to be healthy when all its parts are in their normal condition and are able to perform their work without uneasiness and pain. A healthy person always feels perfectly well. He feels delight in performing his duty and can bear easily troubles both bodily and mental; he is not worried by cares and anxieties as much as an unhealthy man. He gets natural sleep and possesses natural appetites—and he feels pleasure in all the natural functions which he is required to do by Mother-Nature. He does not get easily excited but remains always in a jolly mood—such a state of health is possible only when we keep our blood pure and body clean.

An Unhealthy State

Disease is a perverted state of body or mind caused by errors in diet and by unnatural mode of living. It is the natural consequence of our own wrong actions. That a morbid condition of health is the result of auto-toxin generated from the disorganised substances in the body itself or from the unwholesome non-nutritive foreign substances introduced into the body in the form of food, drink, medicine, vaccines, serums, etc. which as a rule make the body unclean and the blood impure. Uneasiness of mind, irritability, bodily pain, disinclination for mental or physical exertion, inability to do one's own duties, unnatural cravings, want of appetite or sleep, etc. are the symptoms of a morbid condition of health.

How Disease is caused and how it should be remedied

It is a very stupid and sad error to believe that disease is a divine scourge to punish the sins of man. All the diseases in the world are the inevitable consequence of our offences against the laws of Nature in our mode of life.

Every keen observer of Nature knows that good health is the result of implicitly obeying the laws of Nature and disease is the result of transgressing them.

Causes of Disease

Allopathy the ruling medical profession avers that the cause of disease is its bacillus, to destroy which a suitable poisonous drug should be adminstered.

Ayurvedic physicians say :—

व्याधिस्तु दोषवैषम्यं दोषसाम्यमरोगता ॥
तस्मात्स्वास्थ्यं च दोषाणां यत्नतो रक्षयेद् बुधः ॥

Translation :—Disease is the abnormal condition of the humours in the body, while their normal condition constitutes health. Therefore a wise man should always try to keep his humours in their proper conditions.

Unanee Hakims say that :—Red blood, black blood, yellow bile and white phlegm are the important fluids in the body and that health depends on their proper condition.

But a Naturopath says :—

निदानं सर्वरोगाणां विविधाऽहितसेवनम् ॥

"The main cause of all diseases is the unnatural mode of living and chiefly the over taxed condition of the stomach and liver caused by foods not meant by Nature for our consumption. These foods are (1) Artificially manufactured sugar, its preparations, saccharine, etc. (2) Sea-salt, and its preparations, (3) tea, wines, liquors and other stimulating drinks, (4) coffee, tobacco, and other narcotics, (5) fish, fowl, flesh-meat, pork and other animal foods, (6) food-stuffs fried in ghee, oil or fat whether of vegetable, flesh-meat, fish, fowl, etc., or grains such as sweetmeats, *bajyas, chivada,* etc. (7) condiments and their preparations such as spiced milk, cakes, *chutnees,* pickles, etc. (8) preserved food such as jams, jellies, condensed milk, tinned fish, salted bacon, etc. (9) All the crude mineral substances chiefly salts and acids such as chunam eaten with betal-leaf, sea salt, rock salt, epsom salt, glauber's salt, carbonate of soda chiefly in aerated waters, vinegar, tarteric acid, etc. (10) all the poisonous drugs, Opium, Mercury, Arsenic, Aconite, Nux vomica, etc. specially in large doses in mixtures prescribed by medical men whether Ayurvedic, Unanee or Allopathic, are the most objectionable substances to be poured or thrown into our tender stomach.

Air, Water and Sunlight

Man is an animal living essentially on air, Nature has left him on the surface of this Earth surrounded by pure air. So he should spend full 24 hours of the day in fresh air, and he should not lock himself up in rooms where fresh air is not allowed. He should pass his time in sunlight at least from 8 to 12 hours daily, as Nature sheds such light on him daily at least for such a length of time. But he should not be in water more than 20 to 30 minutes at a time. He may be in water for about 60 minutes in a day but not longer. A human being who observes these rules will continue to be healthy without getting ill at all, if he obeys other laws of Nature.

Man transgresses the laws of nature almost every moment, regarding air, water, earth, sunlight, food, sleep, exercise, etc. and consequently he becomes ill. Adolph Just says that only by returning to the harmony in which Nature had originally placed him can he regain his health and be entirely free from disease.

It is quite reasonable and true that if the diseased condition is caused by disobeying the laws of Nature that it will be cured by obeying them only. It is also plain that if a disease cannot be cured by natural methods, it will never be cured by poisons and other unnatural methods; on the contrary it will be made worse by them. It is Nature that cures in spite of them where she gets chances to do so and where there is sufficient vitality left in the patient. **Vis Medicatrix Naturæ.**

What Nature does to restore health in such morbid conditions

Nature the kind mother of all makes every effort to eliminate all poisons from our system in order to keep us healthy. This may be clearly observed in catarrh, cough, fever, night-sweats, haemorrhages, diarrhœa, dysentery, scurvy, pyorrhœa, metrorrhagia, leucorrhœa, eczema, eruptions, boils, carbuncles, ulcers, cancers, etc. Dr. Lindlahr says :—"Every acute disease is the result of the cleansing and healing efforts of Nature."

Dr. Trall says—All morbid actions are evidences of the remedial efforts of Nature to overcome morbid conditions or expel morbid materials. All that any truly philosophical system of medication can do, or should attempt to do, is to place the organism under the best possible circumstances for the favourable operation of those efforts. We may thwart, embarass, interrupt or suppress them as is usually the case with allopathic practice or we may direct, modify, intensify or accelerate them as to the legitimate province of hydropathic practice. But we must admit to the paradoxical proposition that the symptoms of disease are the evidences of the restorative effort; the effort, however may be unequal to the end in view, and hence the powers of Nature are to be assisted in removing obstacles, diverting irritation, etc."

Carrington says "That we must always bear in mind—the fact that all disease is itself a curing process or method of elimination, and, as such, cannot possibly be cured! Thus a cold is merely a process of expelling through the nose impurities that should have been up and eliminated through other more natural channels. A boil is but the same process in operation in a little different way; a cough is merely the effort of

Nature to expel solid material from a locality where it has no right to be; a pain is only a symptom and not a disease at all—merely an indication of such; a fever is simply a natural process of rapid combustion "the burning up" of this material unduly retained within the organism; a night sweat is merely another attempt on the part of Nature to eliminate this material through the skin and so on throughout the list."

Elimination of Poisons Versus Suppression of Disease

Every acute disease is the effort of Nature to cleanse the body of its impurities or morbid matter which is likely to endanger health and life. Hence it is the duty of a physician in such cases to help Nature in getting rid of such impurity, it may be a foreign matter or some disorganised substance of the body. But the medical profession tries to suppress the disease by giving poisons and benumbing the affected parts instead of eliminating those poisons from the body. For instance all fevers are suppressed by Quinine, Antipyretics, Anti-toxins, Serums, etc., but these will paralyse the red and white corpuscles of the blood, weaken the heart and depress all vital functions; pain and sleeplessness are checked by bromides, opiates and sedatives which benumb the brains and nerves; constipation is relieved by strong purgatives which cause more severe types of constipation later on. Diarrhoea and dysentery are checked with opium preparations which paralyse the peristaltic action of bowels or cause obstinate constipation later on. Gonorrhœa is checked by local injectic ıs which may cause orchitis, buboes or rheumatism. Syphilis is checked by cauterisation, mercury, iodine, arsenic, etc., which as a rule cause more serious consequences later on. All nervous diseases are checked by bromides which benumb brain and nerves and cause premature old age, idiocy or paralysis. Skin diseases are suppressed by ointments containing sulphur, zinc, etc., which may cause headache, vertigo, asthma, cataract, insanity, epilepsy, et ., or the same diseases reappear later on with greater severity. Teeth, tonsils, glands, varies, tumours, piles, appendix, etc., are removed when those are affected; but these surgical operations do not remove the cause of these affections and thereby the patient's general health gets more affected later on. Measles, small-pox, chicken pox, etc. if suppressed before they run their proper course, cause serious consequences later on.

Dr. Lindlahr says—"Instead of purifying the human bodies of morbid waste, systemic poisons and disease taints, the medical profession saturates them with drug poisons and disease products, under the guise of medicines, vaccines, serums and antitoxins." It is equivalent to saying, "there is no need of cleaning your house in order to prevent moulds, fungi and vermin. All that is necessary is to deligently soak the premises with antiseptics and germ-killers. Such practice may succeed for a while, but what condition will the house be in, if dirt and poisonous chemicals are allowed to accumulate."

From time immemorial Naturopaths have been curing all kinds of serious acute and chronic diseases with the help of fresh air, pure water and bright sun light without the help of any poisonous drugs.

"Nothing in the world" says Platen "should be of greater concern to a man, nothing should be considered of greater value, than the preservation of health. It should be his most earnest desire to enjoy continuous good health."

All know fully well that Nature alone heals, and that it is the natural power within us which alone can destroy disease ; we must leave it to this power which never errs, and never takes the wrong road to attain its object. That is why it is so dangerous to use all kinds of poisonous medicines which suppress and finally destroy the great gift which cures. Long illness and fatal endings can be the only result of such proceedings."

Many parents are very careful to educate their children in schools and colleges, but they are not so careful to train them up in matters of health and hygiene. An elementary knowledge of sanitation and hygiene should be made compulsory in all the primary schools, as it will teach children how to be free from disease and anxiety. He is really happy whose body is healthy and mind contented. To attain this end we should make it a sacred duty to become fully acquainted with the causation of disease and the natural means of healing the various kinds of it.

"Thousands of persons die yearly for lack of light, air and water which are the very principles of our existence and without which we must sicken and die.

Diseases are increased and made incurable through wrong treatment with poisonous drugs. It is better and safer therefore to treat patients according to law of Nature with her own remedies." (Platen).

One may be able to speak the language of the Romans, Greeks, Britons, French and Germans, and may have studied Physics, Chemistry, Botany, Zoology, etc. and may have mastered Surgery, Materia Medica, Therapeutics, Bacteriology, Dermatology, Embryology, Veneriology, Vaccine therapy, Serum therapy, Electro-therapy, Organo-therapy, etc., but if one has not studied the laws of Nature and not found out the key to her ways one will not be able to prevent nor cure diseases. " Vis Medicatrix Naturæ."

" The language of Nature can be learnt neither in hot-class rooms, nor from the corpse in the disecting room, nor from tortured animals in the laboratory, neither from the sufferers in the hospital. Nature alone can teach us." (Prof. Gustav Jager).

" The future belongs to popular hygiene and to the natural curative system of treatment that is based on the laws of unerring Nature. The natural healing system will spread beyond its present narrow limits and attain a world wide predominance. It has a great social function to perform. It fights against the excessive luxury and refinement of modern life, against drink and dissipation of every kind ; and it does for the individual with its gospel of health what public hygiene seeks to do for community to promote the " health" and the welfare of the people" (M. Platen).

Advantages of Naturopathy

Dr. Korner writes :—

(1) Nature's healing force makes steady progress towards recovery in all diseases if the patient acts according to Naturopathic treatment.

(2) More lives are saved by natural treatment than by medical ; in unfavourable cases at the most four or five out of a hundred are lost where as under medical treatment according to Dr. Schonlein more than 30 per cent. of the favourable cases die.

(3) It leads to a much more speedy recovery of health ; as a rule in severe cases the patient is to be considered convalescent in the fourth week.

(4) It cures the disease thoroughly and effectually so that the blood and the humours are cleared of all morbid matter and no after diseases can arise ; where as medically treated patients often die from these some time afterwards.

(5) It is cheaper since it leads to recover most rapidly and cuts down the doctor's bills without having any chemists' bills at all.

(6) It does not let the disease develop if it is applied as soon as the symptoms are noticed but it cuts it short as is clear from the nature of the treatments which endeavours to purify the blood so as to prevent a localisation of the virus.

(7) Cleanliness is another consideration and the remedies can be had every where as supplied by Nature.

(8) It is more comforting to the relatives of the patient that they do not find the doctor looking grave and shaking his head and shrugging his shoulders but confident about his treatment while under medical treatment consultation after consultation is held, one physic after another is tried all which must fill the unfortunate relatives with care and anxiety. (Platen).

(9) Self-treatment is possible.

(10) There is no confusion in the mode of treatment as it is very simple, and as our own instinct guides us to observe it.

2. Some Pioneers of Naturopathy

The views of **Charaka**, the illustrious founder of the Ayurvedic Medical system and the oldest of the Naturopathic Physicians known and of his followers regarding the use of fresh air, pure water and bright sunlight are as follows :—

वायुरायुर्बलं वायुर्वायुर्धाता शरीरिणाम्
वायुर्विश्वमिदं सर्वं प्रभुर्वायुश्च कीर्तितः
अव्याहतगतिर्यस्य स्थानस्थः प्रकृतौस्थितः
वायुःस्यात्सोऽधिकं जीवेद् वीतरोगः समाः शतम्

(Charaka Part 4–28).

Translation—Air is the life of living beings, air is their strength and air is their sustainer. Air is the cause and all pervading substance of this universe.

In whose body air is allowed to pervade freely in a pure and natural state, he will be able to live for more than a century free from any disease.

पानीयं प्राणिनां प्राणा स्तदायत्तं हि जीवितम्
तस्मात्सर्वास्ववस्थासु वारि देयं पिपासवे
दिवा सूर्यांशुसंतप्तं रात्रौ चंद्रांशुशीतलम्
अंशूदकमितिख्यात मायुरारोग्यदायकम्

Translation—Water is the life of living beings, and their very subsistence depends on water only. Therefore water should be given to the thirsty in whatever condition they may be.

That water which is heated during the day by the rays of the sun and cooled at night time by the lunar beams is called "*Anshoodaka*" It can impart good health and prolong life.

सूर्यातपः स्वेदवहः सर्वरोगविनाशकः
भेदच्छेदकरश्चैव बलोत्साहविवर्धनः

Translation—The sun's rays induce perspiration and cure all diseases. They are also reducers of fat and promoters of vigour and cheerfulness.

दद्रुविस्फोटकुष्ठघ्नः कामलाशोथनाशकः
ज्वरातिसारशूलानां हारको नात्र संशयः

Translation—There is no doubt that they are the healers of ringworm, eruptions, leprosy, anæmia, dropsy, fever, diarrhœa and colic.

कफपित्तोद्भवान् रोगान् वातरोगान् तथैव च
तत्सेवनाच्चरोजित्वा जीवेच्च शरदां शतम्

Translation—By their daily use a man may be able to live for a hundred years, having overcome all ailments caused by the derangements of phlegm, bile and wind.

The daily discipline enjoined by the sages of old was briefly as follows :—

Cold water bath early in the morning followed by 12 salutations to the sun the protector and healer of all diseases. Please see the chapter VIII on breathing for the mode of salutations. The same programme was to be gone through at midday when the sun was at its meridian and again at about sunset.

Thus the advantages of water-bath, sun-bath, air-bath and exercise were secured. In the absence of facilities for any other exercise the number of salutations may be increased to 108 or 120 every time; with advanced age they must be gradually decreased to 12 at a time.

Patanjali the founder of Yoga system of philosophy and his followers have indicated several modes of breathing exercise, (प्राणायाम) and Psycho—physical exercise योगासन and योगमुद्रा—They are very useful both to preserve health and to improve it when it is impaired.

Herodicus and **Democritus** the two famous Greek Physicians of antiquity recommended a Natural curative treatment grounded on systematic exercise and diet. The latter lived for 109 years free from disease. **Hippocrates** who is known as the father of Allopathic Medical Science all over Europe and who lived in the fifth century B C. says, "Naturae sanat, medicus curat." "It is Nature that heals disease. The Physician is to assist her in her healing process." According to him a complete knowledge of all the ways of Nature, of dietic treatment, the use of every form of massage (rubbing) exercise and bath and a knowledge of Astrology were necessary for every physician. He lived 109 years.

Theophrastus Paracelsus a Naturopath and a renowned German alchemist was born in 1494 and died on the 23rd of September 1541. He was an Allopathic M. D.

He combined a vast knowledge of natural science with that of medicine. He was the first to work against the old established theories and it was reserved for him to break down the temptations of the method laid down by Galenus. This revolution by the way was brought about by his researches made for the Philosopher's stone which was supposed to turn baser metals into gold, and for the Elixir of Life which was to prove itself a universal cure. In spite of his failure in these directions he made discoveries which proved of great importance both to medicine and chemistry. His motto was "Natura artis magistra" i. e. Nature is the teacher of science. He was the first to propound the theory of the existence of magnetic properties in the human body.

Hahnemann the founder of Homeopathy who was born in 1755 and died in 1843 was another Allopathic M. D. of Germany. He not only pointed out the errors and dangerous practices in medicine which prevailed in his time but also pointed out the humane and simpler mode of treatment. In 1784 he wrote and published a book on the cure of chronic diseases with water-treatment and massage.

Vincent Priessnitz was a great Pioneer of hydropathic (water-cure) treatment. He was born on the 4th of October 1799. In 1819 he had the misfortune of having his ribs broken by the up-setting of his carriage. He got himself cured by hydropathic treatment after an allopathic doctor had pronounced his case as incurable. Thereafter he tried with remarkable success the same mode of treatment for all the patients who came to him. As the number of his patients increased he built his hydropathic establishment in 1826 at Græfenberg in Austrian Silesia and spent the remaining days of his life in treating the patients free of charge. He had to suffer a good deal at the hands of the allopathic doctors of his time. But he is now styled the father of hydropathic mode of treatment and almost all allopathic doctors now make use of his methods.

Johann Schroth was kicked by a horse in 1817 with the result that his right knee-cap was badly crushed. The limb was treated according to surgical methods, but he remained lame as the cure was incomplete. By making use of cold water compress he got a complete cure. He found that warmth induced by moisture had cured him. So he tried the same measures with a special dietary system on injuries, stiff joints, rheumatism, etc. both among his neighbours and animals and was able to cure them all with wonderful success. During a practice of twenty six years Schroth effected some marvellous cures; some maladies which had defied every kind of medical treatment yielded to his simple procedure; some others which threatened to terminate fatally unless the knife was applied, abated in severity and finally disappeared" (Platen).

Arnold Rikli was born on February 13th 1823 at Veldas in Carniola. He founded the system of treatment of diseases with airbaths and sunbaths according to the principles of Nature.

If water does good, air does more.

The sun does most whom we adore—V. M. Kulkarni.

He regarded them as remedies of the highest order as his motto shows and he rightly called them the simplest and most beneficial means of curing, strengthening and hardening the human body. He teaches us plainly that if we are to benefit by the light and air treatment we must not expose ourselves to the influence of these two agents while we wear clothes, but a light and air bath must be taken in a state of perfect nudity, if it is to have a permanent and beneficial result.

In his treatment of the sick, Rikli employs other natural remedies such as water, diet, exercise, rest, etc. but by his method we understand the application of air and light as remedies for disease. He is the proprietor of a Sanitorium conducted in accordance with these principles. It is situated at Veldas, one of the most beautiful and picturesque regions of the world (Platen).

Light has a very great influence upon vegetable and animal life.—Different rays of solar light have different effects. Vegetable physiology teaches us that the extreme red rays of the solar spectrum convey heat; the yellow rays give nourishment and by means of chlorophil they decompose carbonic acid gas; the blue rays are the cause of movement in the various parts of a plant and so are productive of growth; the extreme violet rays produce blossoms.

Scientists have proved that the skin of animals is sensitive to light and colour; light penetrates not only the outer, but also the inner surface of the skin and this being the case, it follows that it is impossible for animal life to be maintained in health without light and especially without the light of the Sun. In large cities those who live in dark dwellings become pale and anæmic and are subject to many diseases. Every living creature on our planet whether animal or vegetable requires light in order to maintain its health and becomes diseased in the dark. The beneficial influence of light is our reason why it is whole-some to be in the open air, and to be in the light is as important as breathing pure air, rich in oxygen, and taking exercise (Platen). Rikli says "The relative value of light, air and water corresponds to their capacity of acting upon the human body. Light has the greatest capacity and water the least whilst air stands midway between them (Platen).

The patient must have light, but not sit exposed to the sun's rays longer than is needed to bring about welcome warmth. As soon as the sunbath produces restlessness, the person under treatment must move into the shade. If great weakness exists the ordinary amount of clothing must be worn, as strength returns, let the feet be bared up to the ankle, and so on until the whole body bathes as it were on the sun and air (Platen).

Kneipp was a Roman Catholic Priest in Bavaria. He was born in 1824. To quote his own words—"I was broken in body and mind; I myself had given up hope and looked forward with resignation to my end. With Hydropathic treatment I became all right; I gained strength more and more, became a priest and have followed my sacred vocation for thirty-six years." He recommends affusions of cold water in pains and injuries, dipping the parts in tepid water in burns and scalds, enema in constipation and walking bare-footed on the ground or grass in all nervous diseases; his douche bath is an excellent hydropathic treatment in many obstinate complaints, and is now adopted by all the hydropaths in the world. He advised his patients to wear loose clothing so as to ventilate all their pores.

Kuhne's life was saved by hydropathic treatment when he was one foot in the grave and when the allopathic doctors of his time had pronounced that his illness was incurable. He maintains that the cause of all diseases is the presence of foreign matter *i. e.* impurities in the body, which always accumulate in the abdomen and then enter into the blood. In all ailments therefore he recommends the use of steam baths followed by friction hip-baths. The former induces free perspiration and the latter free motions and thus the body is made free from impurities in a very short time. In chronic cases only the treatment is required longer. He maintains that foreign matter and impurities in the body are caused by over-eating or by consuming substances not meant by Nature as our food stuff; for instance flesh-meat, spices, alcohol, narcotics, stimulating drinks, chemicals, drugs, patent medicines, etc., vaccine poison or calf-lymph inserted in the body as a preventive of small-pox and the use of tobacco in the form of chewing, smoking, snuffing, etc, he considers objectionable. He recommends milk, fruits, nuts, cereals, herbs, vegetable and water in all cases of ailments.

"Disease" says **Kuhne** "is the presence of foreign matter in the system". There are two passages through which matter can be introduced into the body by the nose into the lungs, and by the mouth into the stomach. Each of these passages is guarded by sentinels, who are not, however thoroughly incorruptible and sometimes let things pass which do not belong to the body. These sentinels are the nose and the tongue, the one for air and the other for food. As soon as we fail to promptly obey the senses of smell and taste they grow lax in the fulfilment of their duty and gradually allow harmful matter to pass unchallenged into the body, you are aware how one can become used to sitting in dense clouds of tobacco smoke inhaling it just as if it were healthy fresh air. The tongue has been still further corrupted and we know that it can gradually be habituated to a most unnatural food. Need I remind you of the different dishes and beverages which we now think indispensable though they were unknown some centuries ago?"

Prof. Wilhelm Winternitz was born at Josefstadt in Bohemia in 1834. He graduated in medicine in the University of Vienna in 1855 and took his Diploma as a Doctor of Medicine and entered the navy when he was only twent yone years of age. On a warship he had to treat a case of influenza which did not yield to the usual medical treatment; at last he tried water treatment; being gratified with the wonderful result of water he began to study the science thoroughly from the then renowned authors on hydropathy and at last went to Graefenberg to gain practical knowledge.

In 1862 he opened the first Institute of Hydropathy at Kaltinleutgehm near Vienna. It soon became a large Hospital accommodating several hundreds of in-patients with arrangements for several outpatients also. In due course he was appointed Lecturer in Hydropathy at the University of Vienna. He also built an hospital in connection with the poly-clinic where patients were treated with sunbaths and air-baths, diet, massage, etc. He edited a journal called "Blatter Fur Klinische Hydrotherapie" for nineteen years. He completed his learned work "Magnum Opus" in 1879. He has been frequently quoted as one of the best authorities in hydropathy and chromopathy (sunlight cure) by the European and American medical authors.

Pier Henrik Ling (born 1776 and died in 1851) was the originator of hygienic Swedish movements of the limbs. He condemned drug treatment of diseases and showed how his new method of different movements of the limbs without the use of any apparatus could be prophylactic and curative of all ailments. It is he who laid the foundations of the present methods of physical culture and hygienic exercises.

Prof. F. E. Bilz is a strong advocate of the Natural method of healing. He built the Bilz Institution at Dresden-Radebeul in Germany. He is the author of the first Naturopathic Encyclopœdia, the "Natural Method of Healing" and several other works on Natural Life and Nature cure.

Dr. Katz Surgeon-in Chief of the Prussian Army was another staunch advocate and practitioner of the

Natural Healing Method. He founded a Nature-cure-Sanitorium at Hoehenwaldau-Degerloch near Stuttgart, Germany. He worked as a director there till his death.

Dr. H. Lahmann is another staunch advocate of Naturopathy. When he was expelled by the university of Leipzig for spreading so-called medical sedition, he was obliged to go to Switzerland to finish his medical education. He founded a Nature-cure Institution at Weisser Hirsch near Dresden in Saxony. He was the author of several books on Diet, Nature-cure and Heliotherapy. The present Biochemic system of Medicine of Dr. Schuessler is the development of his work entitled "*Nutritive Salt Theory*". He denounced drug-treatment as unscientific and harmful and strongly advocated the use of "*light and air*".

Adolph Just is a strict observer of the Laws of Nature. His work "Return to Nature" has been translated into all the European languages. It was he who founded the original "Jungborn" Natural Healing Institute of Germany.

Edwin D. Babbitt of America was a great pioneer of Chromopathy or Heliotherapy. In his masterly work entitled "The Principles of light and colour" published in 1878, he has distinctly shown that with the help of light and colours it is possible to cure even so called incurable diseases. He distinctly states that an ignorant healer who deals with the finer forces of Nature will in most cases do more good and less harm to his patients than a so called learned physician who practises only with the coarser elements.

Dr. Carl Strueh, is one of the most eminent medical men who preferred the Natural mode of treatment to medical practice and surgery in America. He established in 1897 the first drugless Institute in Chicago. There he freely made use of air bath, sun bath, water applications, out-door life, systematic curative exercise, massage and natural diet.

Mr. Tukaram Tatya Fellow of the Theosophical Society of Bombay was a strong advocate of Homœopathy and Naturopathy. The author was an eye-witness to more than a hundred wonderful cures which he had achieved between 1890 and 1900 where leading Allopathic and Ayurvedic Physicians of his time had failed. In all nervous diseases as a rule he tried Mesmerism and in all other cases Chromopathy and Homœopathy. Like Dr. Lindlahr of America he used to say that Homœopathy was in accordance with Nature's laws.

Dr. V. M. George of Columbus, Ohio, has been a practising Physician, since 1866. Although 84 years of age, he looks as if still on the sunny side of sixty. He is a staunch and loyal advocate of natural living and healing. He is a living example of what he believes and teaches. He is a very kind-hearted man; his sympathy and help are extended to every worthy cause. (Herald of Health October 1920).

Miss Jessie Allen Fowler, Deen of the new York phrenological Institute is another advocate of drugless healing and natural living.

Mrs. Diana Belais Editor of the "Open Door", Founder and president of the Anti-Vivisection Society of America is a champion of drugless therapy She is rendering valiant service to this humanitarian cause through her magazine " Open Door. "

Mary Nichols an English lady who fully believes in the natural mode of treatment, and who condemns drug treatment says " Every considerate person will admit that it is the first duty of a physician not to interfere with the healing powers of Nature. If he can't improve the condition of the patient, he should not at least make it worse. All that can be safely done by a physician is to aid Nature in her work of healing as she is the greatest of the healers. But this is not to the interest of druggists and practitioners of drug-system and their mode of treatment of diseases is always thwarting the progress of Nature while the water-cure treatment is a scientific application of the principles of Nature in the cure of disease. It cleanses the system by removing the morbific matter from the body and invigorates it without making use of any drastic measures. "

Trall, Wilson, Rev. Strœbele, Kellogg, Lindlahr, Kipnis, Lust and MacFadden in America have made their names immortal by condemning treatment with poisonous drugs and recommending Nature's bounties as the best medium for the preservation of health and also for recouping it.

3. A Brief Auto-Biography of the Author.

I was born in a village called Bankikodla in North Canara District. Both of my parents were quite healthy; they needed no medicine at all till they breathed tneir last. My father was 85 years old when he died and my mother was 70 years old when she died ; she being ten years younger than my father. I was bright and healthy, till I was vaccinated.

After vaccination, I became unhealthy, irritable, rickety and troublesome to the dissatisfaction of my parents and relatives. They tried their best to improve my condition but failed. They consulted Allopathic doctors and Ayurvedic physicians and kept me under their treatment but without any improvement. My health got worse day by day and I became a wreck and a cause of anxiety to my parents. Still I was attending an Anglo-vernacular school in that village and I was an object of pity of all those who took interest in me especially as I kept up a high rank in the class. My thread ceremony was performed later than usual merely as a necessary religious ceremony without the usual eclat.

As my parents were very nervous about my poor health they would not send me away from them for the prosecution of higher studies. At last I came to Bombay with a friend of mine against their will. I was shown to several allopathic doctors ; they drugged me for some time and said that my case was a peculiar one and suggested little hope of recovery.

At last Mr. Tukaram, a Homœopath and a Naturopath and a Fellow of the Theosophical Society gave me some hopes and cured me with a few doses of high potencies of *Thuja* and *Silicea.* I was also told to take cold water baths and morning walks in bright sunlight daily. This remarkable incident prompted me to study Homœopathy and Naturopathy myself and give the advantage of my studies and experience to the suffering.

From ill effects of vaccination fell
I turned a hopeless wreck and was unwell
Then purged with nostrums and drugs infernal
I did lose faith in all unnatural
And sought for health on Nature's mount and field
Which sunshine bright with ozone daily yield
Fresh air, pure water, ripe fruits and bright light
Were Nature's free gifts that set me all right.
Since then for health on Nature I depend
And never take drugs noxious health to mend
By making free use of these gifts sublime
I can keep up my health in any clime.
The blessing of good health you can enjoy
Great Nature's kind gifts if you do employ
Both to preserve and to restore your health
Which you can do without expending wealth
This I say and assure you, readers dear
You can all practise and make it quite clear
All drugs and poisons in our blood diffuse
And serious harm is caused by their use
V. M. Kulkarni hence you doth implore
Kind Nature's wholesome food-store to explore
And to avoid all drug and poison store
As it is not meant in your throat to pour.

My parents who had at one time thought my days were numbered had the satisfaction to see me hale and hearty and an earning member of the family and also a father of eight healthy children (seven sons and a daughter).

Copy of the circular issued by the author

Vis Medicatrix Naturæ.

Since 1889 I have been not only treating patients gratis on **Naturopathic** principles with remarkable results, but also training students free of charge.

The principles of **Naturopathy** are :—

1. A healthy human body does not contain any poisons in it.

2. Human beings do not get ill if they lead a natural life and take no poisons in their system.

3. They need no poisons to get cured when they get ill.

4. If blood is kept pure and vitality preserved, they continue to be healthy; even if they inhale millions of microbes, the disease germs will perish as they cannot thrive in pure blood.

5. But if the blood gets impure even a single microbe will propagate millions of its species in the human bodies; nay, even if they do not inhale a single disease germ they will get some disease, with innumerable microbes peculiar to that disease, as microbes are the scavengers of wise Nature.

In such cases:—

Fresh air, pure water and bright light
With proper food will set us right.
And in fact there is not a need
Of any poisonous drugs indeed.

All diseases even so called incurable ones can be treated successfully with fresh air, pure water, bright light and Nature's food supply. No drugs, no poisons, no injections, nor any unnatural drastic measures are needed in the treatment of diseases according to Naturopathy. Since 1919 arrangements have been made to train students in Elementary Anatomy, Physiology, Hygiene, Sanitary Science, etc., in the Bombay Homœpathic Medical College, Princess Street. I have been instructing the students of the said college in Naturopathy also without any charge. Whoever wishes to study this important Healing Art in all its branches may apply to the undersigned. Diploma of merit is supplied to the successful students.

Do study Nature's Mystery
From ailments as she makes us free,
Though frequently we disobey
Her laws and take drugs every day.

V. M. KULKARNI,
Homœopath & Naturopath,
C/o Roy & Co., Homœopaths
Princess Street, Bombay, India.

* * * *

How I keep fit and what I do to combat disease

I daily rise in morn at six
And at once the day's programme fix
Thus when I leave my nightly bed
With my own hands I rub my head
And body till they all aglow
And they feel warmth from top to toe
Then I wash my eyes and the top
Of head at once without a stop
Sit under pipe or in a tub
And my whole body fast I rub

By bathing thus in water cold
I feel refreshed a thousand-fold
If I miss by chance tub and pipe
I take a bath of ancient type
By pouring on head water pure
To drench the body and secure
A bath complete to cleanse the skin
And by brisk rubbing a glow within ;
That plenty water clean and fresh
Doth my mind and body refresh.

I bathe in summer twice a day
But only once in winter's sway
In regions hot I bathe three times
But only once in colder climes.

In rainy season at least thrice
Rain bath I take above all price

For nerves it doth electrify
And body too re-vivify.;
A shower bath on head and spine
And neck is a good plan of mine
All won'drous benefit of rain
From shower bath we can obtain
For it prevents neuralgic pain
And from it one can vigour gain
It stimulates the withered skin
By quickening the blood within
These showers when streamed on the head
Like soothing balm cure all pains dread.
To my skin I do not apply
Scents, perfumes or oils scented high
Nor I use any scented soap
Nor with such fashions try to cope
Nor otto strong I like to smell
Such products make me feel unwell
Aroma of the flowers sweet
And fragrance of ripe fruits I greet.

Soon after bath light exercise
And rest I take in happy wise
A cup of fresh milk then I sip
Eat some fruits and start for a trip
Or tender cocoanut I eat
Crammed with both food and drink so sweet
I prefer it to milk and fruits
Uncommonly my health it suits
In countries hot it is a boon
Of Nature to quench our thirst soon.

Then I take a walk decked in white
In gardens bathed in solar light
Where creepers tender, carpets green
And blossoms blooming beckoning seen
Where whistling winds the trees bend low
And with their fragrance ceaseless blow
Where plants all glisten with drops of snow
Which shine like pearls in morning glow
Where creepers cling to trees all day
Though they by winds are blown astray
Where transitory charms are shown
By flowers when they are full blown
Where noble trees with their fruits bend
As if their harvest rich to lend—
To all those who would be in need
Like charitable men indeed
Where some plants sing with hissing sound
And others bend to kiss the ground
Where cuckoos black sing their sweet song
And they allure my mind there long
Where humming bees keep lingering
And little birds keep chir-ruping
As if they Nature's praises sing
And heartily thank blooming spring
Where golden rays of morning light
Instill new life and pure delight
I walk along with wondering sight
Till all my limbs are tired out right
In rounds of daily exercise
We can draw much from Nature wise.

At half past ten my meal I eat
Of wholesome fruits and nuts and wheat,
I loathe fish, fowl and flesh as meat
And don't allow them near my seat
I don't eat eggs nor custard sweet
These on my table I don't greet
No pudding sweet, nor any cake
Nor biscuits nor fried things I take
I don't take hodge-podge, pastry, cheese
Nor any substance mixed with grease
I don't like salt nor salted food
As they cause thirst and do no good
Both *chutneys*, pickles I do hate
To eat spiced things I hesitate
As they did always constipate
My bowels when those things I ate
I don't like jams and sweetmeats grand
Their taste and smell I cannot stand
For pungent things I have dislike
And foods preserved I seldom like
Hence take nuts and fruits quite a lot
But never eat things cold or hot
As neither of them ever serve
Our health and vigour to conserve
Refreshed then I attend my work
Week in week out not known to shirk
My second meal I take at five
Of fruits and nuts and thus I thrive
With a cup of milk fresh and pure
Toil and fatigue I can endure.

This simple life I always live
As peace and joy naught else can give.
At half past five I take again
A pleasant walk health to retain
On pleasant hill side or green field
Or on beach which fresh air rich yield
At nine P. M. I never sup
But only drink a sober cup
Of cocoa-water, fruit juice fresh
Or Adam's ale which does refresh
I keep awake till ten to read
Then go to bed for sleep I need
By keeping windows open at night
For fresh air I sleep till morn bright.
Whenever I dont get fresh air
I feel as if in great despair
Hence I don't stand near frying pans
Or flour mills, or motor vans
Near persons with obnoxious itch
Near dung hills or foul smelling ditch
Or engine in which workers stoke
Or furnace giving out much smoke
Near stagnant ponds I never stop
Or foul fish store or butcher's shop
Or gents or ladies when they smoke
Tobacco in its varied cloak.
I take an air bath twice a day
With one cloth and all dress away
They give me always comfort great
Keep my skin in a healthy state

When daily walks in morn I take
I breathe through nostrils not to stake
My health by breathing through the mouth
The high way for bacilli's growth
In fresh air charged with sunlight bright
I draw deep breaths and feel all right
In breathing I expand my chest
Fresh vigour to get and feel the best
I do first shut up my nostril right
And then inhale till I tire slight
By nostril left and then expel
All the dead cells exhaling well
Then by right nostril I inhale
By shutting left and then exhale
At least ten times thus I breath deep
By habit this my health I keep.
Though parched with great thirst I do not
Quaff, soda, tea, or coffee hot
Or other sweet drinks cooled with ice
Which have become a favourite vice
As they do cause dyspepsia
Or prickly heat or nausea
Or toothache bad or gum's disease
And our heat normal they decrease
As bad is fruity syrup sweet
So a ripe juicy fruit I eat
Drink cocoa-water which gives peace
Or eat a water-melon's piece
Or sugar-cane's which works as well
For quenching thirst they act like spell.

Pipe-water though fresh I do not drink
Well-water makes me with horror shrink
The latter is not touched by sun
The former chlorinated one
E'en butter-milk I do not take
As it's of artificial make
I don't take sherry nor tokay
As these things do not mak me gay
Nor do I take champagne nor wine
Nor liquors which health undermine
I never smoke before my meal
Nor after as I giddy feel
I do not use tobacco snuff
Nor any stupefying stuff
Such as cocaine, opium
Nor things which cause delirium
That betel-nut I never chew
With chunam, leaves and catechu
I never eat boiled and spiced food
Which in no way will do me good
Kind Nature's bountiful supply
Doth both please me and gratify
She is providing for us all
Her sweet foods always natural

Whenever I do not perspire
I stand in the sun and respire
Take deep breaths freely and exhale
These sun baths always keep me hale
Twice in a month I do observe
A partial fast health to conserve

On those days I do only eat
A cocoanut or plantain sweet
That too but once in the fore noon
These fasts I find a saving boon.
I do attend great Nature's call
Without postponing it at all
As habit such would do me harm
And in the long run cause alarm
In noon I don't take a nap light
Nor do I keep awake at night
As Nature has meant night for rest
And day for work and that the best
By strict response to Nature's law
Which I obey with loving awe
And with these good plans every day
I always keep disease away.

My dearest place on earth to me
My heaven on earth I long to see
Is my sweet home where I feel best
And after toil where I take rest
Where I see bright and happy face
Which blooms like lotus from sun's rays
On my return in vig'rous state
And which keeps looking at me straight
Where children young keep frolicking
And servants old keep murmuring
Where rubbish all is cleanly swept
And useful ones in order kept
Where all the guests and beggars too
Do always get their comforts due

Where Nature's gifts have their full scope
With fashions no one tries to cope
All are blessed with simplicity
And natural activity
By easy habits all are true
To their own words and actions too
Where all are strange to lies and fraud
And to the fashionable gaud
Where god of light spreads his bright rays
And whence one can see the moon's grace
For loss sustained where no one wails
Contentment and peace where prevails
That place I find as palace small
Which gives me peace and comforts all.

CHAPTER II

Naturopathy versus Drug Treatment and Drastic Measures.

From time immemorial treatment of disease with poisonous drugs has been condemned by thoughtful men in all countries. But it is still carried on by the medical profession with ever increasing zeal because it is a lucrative method. Both chemists and physicians get rich by trade in these poisons, as the general public is ignorant of their ill-effects. Surely, in these days of much lauded civilization of the twentieth century we are still groping in the medical dark age.

The following verses are found in old Sanskrit literature with special reference to the poison-dealing Vaidyas of that time.

वैद्यराज नमस्तुभ्यं । यमराज सहोदर ॥
यमस्तु हरति प्राणन् । त्वंच प्राणान् धनानि च. ॥

Translation—Oh physician! Salutation to you; (you are) the brother of Yama, (the King of hell). Yama (Your brother) deprives us of our lives only; while you (take away) both our lives and our wealth.

मार्कंडेयो दिवं याति त्वया यदि चिकित्सितः
अरोगोऽपि चिरंजीवी वैद्य दूरान्नमोस्तुते

Translation—Salutation to you Oh physician! from a distance. Even Markandeya though free from disease and blessed with long life hastens to heaven if treated by you.

भिषक् प्रकाशमान् सूर्यो जान्हवीजलमौषधम्
हरिर्हरति रोगांश्च वैद्यो हि यमकिंकरः

Translation—Sun, the God of light is the true physician and the water of the Ganges the true medicine. God Hari cures diseases, while the Vaidya is a servant of Yama (the god of hell).

वैद्यो यमस्य भ्राताऽस्ति दूतो वा मित्रमेव च
गदार्तो मुञ्चति प्राणान् तस्यैवौषधसेवनात्

Translation—The Vaidya is a brother of Yama (the God of hell) or else his messenger or friend. An ailing man dies after taking his medicine.

We may fill volumes with cases under Allopathic practice in which patients lost their lives or suffered seriously; we recommend the book entitled "Medical Crime and Chaos" by an eminent Allopathic doctor of America for the perusal of our readers.

Dr. Foote, M. D., a distinguished allopathic physician of America cites an instance of a young healthy well-built respectable lady. She had two suitors, one of them was a military officer and the other an allopathic doctor. When asked by her mother whom she would prefer she said "neither because both are the killers of mankind one with his weapons and the other with his drugs"—; and she preferred a kind hearted poor school-master. Mr. Gadkari in his well-known drama in Marathi called *"Ekach pyala"* (only one cup) describes a scene near the death-bed of Taleeram. In a dispute between an Allopathic doctor and an Ayurvedic Physician, the former remarks that the patients of Vaidyas (Ayurvedic physicians) as a rule die because the latter cannot diagnose cases well and do not know Bacteriology, etc., while the latter retorts that the patients of Allopathic doctors always die of the poisonous effects of their medicines administered to destroy microbes of the disease and the patients' sons die of heart failure when they see the exorbitant bills presented by doctors after the death of their patients.

There are several similar humorous stories current among the general public about doctors dealing in poisonous drugs. Newspapers report almost daily cases of disastrous results following on the use of poisons. Considerations of space will not permit me to do more than quote a few observations of eminent doctors against the use of poisonous drugs.

1. Dr. Trall says :—" Whatever can be converted into living tissue in the body is food and whatever cannot be done is poison. In a strict sense everything which is not a food is poison. Drugs and medicines of all kinds whether derived from the animal, mineral or vegetable kingdom are poisons and nothing else." " To give drugs is adding to the cause of disease. Indeed, they cure one disease, when they cure at all, by producing others. Can causes cure causes? Can poisons expel poisons? Can impurities deterge impurities? Can Nature throw off two or more burdens more easily than one? No! Poisoning a person because he is diseased is neither scriptural nor philosophical."

2. If one compares the permanent good which half a dozen true sons of Aesculapius have established

on earth since the birth of their art with the evil which an untold number of doctors of this profession have brought on the human race, one is forced to the conclusion that it would have been better for humanity if there had never been any doctors in the world (Dr. Boerhave).

3. There undoubtedly exist very widespread discontent with the so called regular or old allopathic system of medicine. Both here (America) and in Europe a general want of faith in physicians and their art is greatly felt. The cause is palpable; an erroneous theory and injurious, often and very often, destructive exercise of the profession. An intelligent community can only be satisfied by a system of medicine based on reason, in harmony with the infalliable laws of Nature (Prof. Trall)

4. "The medical practice of our day is at best a most uncertain and unsatisfactory system; it has neither philosophy nor common sense." (Dr. Evans)

5. Drugs are uncertain, unsatisfactory and unworthy of confidence. The young practitioner may bear in mind that patients are more often damaged than helped by promiscous drugging. (Dr. Osler).

6. In a large proportion of cases treated by physicians the disease is cured by Nature and not by them; In a lesser but not a small proportion the disease is cured by Nature in spite of them. (Dr. Forbes M. D., F. R. S.).

7. Medicine as now practised is a pestilence to mankind. It has carried off a greater number of victims than all the murderous wars have ever done. (Dr. Hansen Kruger).

8. Medical science is a barbarous jargon, and the effects which our medicines produce on the human system are in the highest degree uncertain; only one thing we are sure of, viz., that they have destroyed more lives than war, pestilence and famine taken together (Dr. J. M. Good).

9. The old saying is, in many cases, true, that physic often does more harm than the malady, and the remedy is worse than the disease. A great many disorders are simply cured by Nature, and the only thing which a physician can and may do in most diseases is to keep off and remove injurious influences, and to abate the abnormal activity of the individual. If he does more, whether to satisfy his patient's craving for medicine, to support his own dogmas, or even to fill his pocket, he can only do mischief. Thus artificial diseases are frequently created, and in many cases of medical treatment it may be maintained that chronic sequelae are produced by the doctor's fault alone, and for that reason every patient should, in consideration of the present state of practical pharmacology, be warned against a doctor as against the most dangerous poison (Dr. Keiser).

10. Professor Dr. Wunderich. well-known in medical schools all over the continent, once declared in

writing that the poisons dealt out by the chemist as remedies are not remedies at all; we should rather learn the use of some non-poisonous plants from shepherds and old women (from Platen).

11. Our medical schools are not centres of progress and enlightment. In spite of all their scientific apparatus, their chemical, pharmaceutical, bacteriological, and physiologcal laboratories their lecture halls and their discoveries they tend to increase the superstition and stupidity of the masses and exist solely to secure the supremacy of a caste condemned as exercising an injurious influence by Petrarch, Ulrich Von Hulten and a great number of honourable and intelligent writers on medicine (Platen).

12. Dr. Carry says—"In the treatment of disease the use of anything not a constituent of the blood is unnecessary; and to give poisons to sick person is simply barbarous and inhuman. True, many have survived it, but equally many have been hurried thus to their graves."

13. The value of medicine expressed in a few words consists principally in the fact that civilised nations have to suffer far more from doctors than from diseases (Dr. Wadekind).

14. A Doctor fond of giving drugs should not came near my sick bed (Prof. Dr. Boch).

15. The whole study of medicine is only an experimental science, we must strive to heal by natural means. We may learn a good deal from old

women and farmers who work their cures with natural methods or by the use of some harmless plants (Prof. Volkmann.).

16. Dr. Densmore says :—Drugs are the shot and shell hurled at the invisible enemy (disease) in the hope of dislodging and expelling it.

17. I fearlessly assert that in the most cases the patient would be more safe without a physician than with one (Prof. Dr. Ramage M. D. F. R. S.).

18. Natural treatment is much more certain to ensure health than a shopful of pharmaceutical poisons" (Platen).

19. The doctor with his medicine has been, is, and will be a necessary and inevitable failure (Lovel).

20. Blumer, a famous Naturopath of America says—" It is better to die a natural death than die of the effects of poisonous drugs; if natural methods of healing fail we are sure the poisonous system will certainly not save such a case, on the contrary it will do some harm; more persons die from drugs than from the original disease."

21. Just as doctors ignorant of the real nature of disease are only able to suppress it and that at the risk of evil results to the system, some surgical operations are performed without sufficient gasp of the vitality of the body which is considered in the light of a machine on which isolated repairs can be made when required. We know now how falacious is this view of things. Hand in hand, too, with the quite evitable

operations there comes the antiseptic treatment for the prevention of mortification. At a Berlin Medical Congress on January 21st 1884 these words were spoken : "Professor Buchner considers the use of antiseptic remedies harmful, for they act more powerfully as poisons on the tissues than on the resisting fungi." Carbolic acid, salicylic acid, iodoform, permanganates, iodides, bromides, sublimate, resorcine, creosote, chloral, etc. ; one making room for the other until yet another took its place.

22 We note that among animals in the natural state the greatest injuries and wounds are effectively healed in an astonishingly short time. An animal in the forest sometimes has a leg shot off or torn away by a trap ; the wound heals completely in a very short time, and the animal continues to live on as if nothing serious had happened. Hence abo[illegible] *and in all cases let us abjure the use of the knife and the scapel on the human body cutting and operating is the crassest contradiction with the processes of Nature and is always followed by the most serious consequences although they may not always manifest themselves at once.* Who ever thinks that it is not always possible to get along without the knife and the scapel, ought in serious cases first try all the means which Nature offers and *these in the right proportion and form* (A. Just)

23. Dr. Tilden of Denver writes in philosophy of Health May 1921 :—The medical profession is as far from the truth today as it was fifty years ago. For proof of this allow me to refer to the daily practice of

our medical school inspectors in prescribing the removal of tonsils and adenoids. Another absurdity being practised daily is that of clearing the mouth of teeth on the pretext of curing rheumatism and other diseases. Women are stripped of their ovaries to cure diseases which could have been cured by medication. Appendix, gall-bladder and other abdominal organs are removed on the pretext that they are a cause of suffering which a correct diagnosis would have traced to gastric and intestinal derangements. (H. H. June 1921).

24. "Sometimes professional zeal, sometimes ignorance and sometimes the prospect of a big fee leads a doctor to undertake an operation" '(H. S. Gray, the Forum May 1915).

Instances of cases of operation under the most skilful and competent hands that have ended in death and dismal failure are not few on record. Several of these cases would not have found grave their early destination had they been treated with natural methods —which ensure cure and invite no possibility of a fatal catastrophe.

Vaccination

"Vaccination is the artificial smallpox caused by inserting some pus into the blood of a healthy person. This pus they scrape out of the running sore of a calf made to suffer from small pox. "This inoculation was based upon the assumption (since known and proven to be false) that any one who had once suffered from small pox could never take it again, and thus if matter from a mild case of smallpox were inoculated upon a healthy child so as to give him small-pox in a mild form, the patient having thus had the disease would be safe from all future contagion." (Foulds).

Dr. D. V. Beacock says that Jenner was not the discoverer of vaccination; he merely revamped an old superstitious bit of folk-lore which enabled him to wheedle the English Government out of 150,000 Dollars (£30,000) through the influence of some of his friends who were then members of the Parliament. He retired on these ill-gotten gains, but the interested parties now manage to keep up their silly fetish alive by muzzling the press, suppressing facts, juggling figures, and deceiving the ignorant public. The idea that a person who had cowpox would not take smallpox was a common legend among the poor ignorant Gloucestershire milking girls and dirty stable boys long before Jenner was born, and in conformity with this beyond the artificial production of cowpox, in order to protect against small-pox, was practised on his own family by an old farmer named Jesty some 20 years before Jenner proclaimed his discovery. Jenner happened to see a milkmaid named Sarah having had some eruptions resembling those of small-pox on her hands and skin; she was actually suffering from secondary syphilis, the eruptions of which resemble those of small-pox in some respect, when questioned by Jenner she told him that she got that infection from the cow's udder while milking a cow ! Jenner was neither a doctor nor a scientist to judge rightly of the case. He was shrewd, stratagic and full of artifice. It was quite natural on the part of Sarah to tell him so to hide the true cause of her disease acquired by immoral actions, and it was also natural on the part of Jenner a non-medical man who had already heard the old folk-lore and what the old farmer Jesty had done, to believe her story and get an inspiration that the artificial small-pox or cowpox would serve as prophylactic for the epidemic form of small-pox.* From these circumstances he not only assured himself that vaccination would serve as a mild form of small-pox which would serve as a prophylactic for further attacks, but he had also the audacity to proclaim that a person once vaccinated is protected for life from small-pox.

But whenever the epidemic of small-pox visited any towns it was found that the first attack was among the vaccinated. It was then decided by the followers of Jenner that a person should be vaccinated once in every ten years. As the condition did not improve even then the period was reduced to seven, then to three and now there are some doctors and vaccinators who advocate that if a person expects to be immune from small-pox he should be vaccinated every year !

But, in spite of vaccination being made compulsory and in spite of entire nations being thoroughly and completely vaccinated out-breaks of small-pox epidemics take place just the same. If at all the attacks and mortality are decreased it is due to the cleanliness and sanitation observed in these days.

---

*The former has a similarity to the latter and Jenner discovered vaccination after the exposition of Homoeopathic law by Hahnemann which also very likely gave him a hint in coming to that conclusion.

Mr. Andrew Eadie, a high authority on sanitation once stated that sanitation, and not vaccination was the real preventive of small-pox.

Alfred Russell Wallace who had watched cases carefully among the vaccinated and nonvaccinated says :—" vaccination is a gigantic delusion. It has never saved one single life. On the contrary, it has caused much suffering and many deaths."

Herbert Spencer has declared that :—vaccination is not only useless but is savage.

Dr. Bell of London says that the principal cause of cancer is vaccination.

The cases of cancer and pyorrhoea were very rare among the higher classes before vaccination was made compulsory by the Government in India.

" Let him that's filthy be so still
Let others be clean if they will "

"Why should a healthy child, perfect from the hands of its creator, be compelled by law to have its pure blood poisoned with rotten (glycerinated or otherwise) pus from the festering sore of a diseased calf, to prevent it taking a possible, but altogether improbable disease—small-pox. " (Dr. D. V. Beacock, Brook Ville Canada).

Dr. Gifford, an American writer, addressing the International Congress in Paris in 1889 used these words :—" To Edward Jenner a great monument in memory has been erected and upon its columns in future, if not in the present, generations will inscribe:—*Accursed be the man by whose cunning devise the blood of all nations has been poisoned.*" It is not only criminal but also sinful to introduce any poison into the stomach or blood of any living being which is likely to do some harm directly or indirectly, sooner or later.

Pus, virus, serum, vaccine fine
Are poisons which health undermine
Fresh air, pure water, sun's bright light
And ripe fruits can keep it all right.

Plague

When the bubonic plague was raging in Bombay (1896–1908) almost every inhabitant was either tempted or forced to get himself inoculated as a preventive measure. Out of those who submitted to inoculation some got mutilated for life and some hurried to an early grave. The enthusiasm of the doctors employed on plague duty was so great that their tongues were always proclaiming the so-called prophylactic efficacy of the serum, as those doctors who praised the serum much and who inoculated a large number received a title of honour from Government for doing their duty properly. Sometime after the news reached in Bombay that a curative serum was being prepared by Dr. Haffkine. From the very news of its preparation both the profession and the laity got delighted and welcomed the day on which it was to be ready and received in Bombay which was then a plague-stricken city. But the serum proved worse than useless as no authenticated case is reported to have been cured by it. Those patients only who were made to live in huts where bright sunlight was penetrating and purifying the air recovered slowly and steadily without any curative injection or poisonous mixture. Sunlight with proper cleanliness is the best prevention and cure for plague. Pure water medicated in bright sunlight by keeping it in blue coloured bottles has cured some cases of plague wonderfully. (See Practical Chromopathy by the author.)

Salvarsan

"Salvarsan is a mixture known as Dianimo-dihidroxyl-arseno benzine-hydro-chloride containing about 31·5 per cent of arsenic metal. Ehrlich himself first claimed that one injection was sufficient to effect a complete cure of syphilis, but actual experience demonstrated later that this was not true so that a series of injections were advised later. And now to make sure of a cure, to the salvarsan, mercury must be added and the latter taken for some few years."

"When the discovery of "606" was flashed round the world several years ago, the claim made for it was utopian. One injection would completely sterilize the system destroying every sperochete or organism of syphilis in the body. After a while it was agreed that two doses were more certain for a thorough cure. Later on some physicians advocated that three to six doses were required to complete the cure. By and by, the number of doses was considerably increased to eradicate the disease."

"Still later when this old, "606" was found useless to cure syphilis radically and was found to result in harmful after-effects the clever german medical statagem brought it up to 914 and now claims that it possesses all the virtues of the old remedy without the ill effects and drawbacks of the old "606," (Dr. Ferri, N. D., Herald of Health—March 1821).

Doctors Boericke and Dewey of America say :—

"A wise Daniel may yet prepare a remedy from measles, cholera or scarlet fever germs which will be just as worthless and perhaps as harmful as Tuberculin of Koch and the antihydrophobic virus of the French Pasteur, with which not only does he seek to cure hydrophobia, but even epilepsy. Pasteur who was a celebrated chemist but no physician, was ignorant of pathology and therapeutics and reminds one, of the tailor of Louis XIV who one day handed to that monarch a memorial on the condition of domestic economy and internal politics. It is self evident that one must be well-versed in anatomy, physiology, pathology and therapeutics and also natural mode of healing disease if one is to become a successful healer. Epilepsy has no similarity what-so-ever with hydrophobia, hence it is more absurd to try to cure epilepsy with hydrophobia-virus than trying to cure syphilis with small-pox or cow-pox virus, or trying to cure any sort of skin disease with "606." Koch's tuberculin may, in some cases effect some favourable changes (to a slight extent for some period) in certain affections of short or long duration but no cure and in many cases aggravations are produced by it shortening the patient's life."

That favourable change or the apparent improvement may be due to the destruction of bacilli caused by the poisonous doses of tuberculinum which may show decrease of fever and cough; but so long as the impurities from the blood, the very soil for the bacilli are not removed and the blood is not oxygenated properly a new growth of tubercular bacilli is sure to take place and send the patient already weakened by the poisonous effects of inoculation to an early grave.

A Naturopath whose treatment consists in the purification of blood finds greater difficulty in treating such a patient as he has to remove not only the original impurities but also the extra virus thus needlessly introduced into the blood.

"When Dr. Koch of Germany announced his remedy now called Kochine, thousands of physicians from all parts of the world, too ready to appreciate the coarse and crude rushed to him. It was thought that it would prove useful in some cases; but the numerous funerals that its use caused in the hospital has laid it mainly on the shelf." (Dr. Babbitt).

Doctors and Quacks

Dr. Schweninger, one of the most celebrated Allopathic doctors says—"The medical profession is losing its prestige and any thinking person must know why. We ourselves are mostly at fault. But the driver curses the bad road if he upsets his cart when drunk; the child beats the table against which it has bumped its head and the doctor blames the "quack" who robs him of the esteem of men."

"We read daily articles of anger and warning as to the ways of wise women; constant accounts appear of the evils wrought by incorrect diagnosis; yet patients consult the "quacks" and men like Kuhne and Gossel have the most important practices in the Kingdom."

"How is this? Are people really so foolish that they think the quack cleverer than the doctor? Surely not; where there is a choice between sour cheap wine and damaged champagne we choose the former and in the same way the person whom the doctor has deceived goes to the quack.

"The mockery of prescriptions is so obvious the chemist alone believes in them now, for his faith is in his income; patients know that there is quackery in the "profession" and that they would rather trust themselves to the quack who follows the dictates of Nature and to Homœopathy rather than to the apothecary's (poisonous) mixtures prescribed by Diplomaed Doctors."

"When Muller senior dies Dr. Crow says that he was wrongly treated by Dr. Smith; but then the latter can tell how Dr. Crow used cold water frictions for Mrs. Werner who was consumptive. So long as medical men put into practice the old saying of the pot calling the kettle black, it is natural that patients will go to quacks and that the latter will write them all down as—fools. And it is we who thus drive the public to quacks."

"Who now is the quack? What right have we to persecute any other medical practitioner as if he were a murderer? Who instituted the water treatment? Priessnitz, a quack; who originated hygienic gymnastics? Ling.

a quack; "how about these and all the other quacks who caused the lame to walk, cured women's diseases which were considered incurable by us and taught us all about massage and muscular exercise? Priessnitz, Hessing, Ling, Wolf, Brand, Kneipp and Thomas will leave their mark indelible in the history of the Art of healing even long after our most celebrated names have been forgotten."

"Despised Homœopathists have proved that patients need not swallow the contents of a chemist's shop (poisonous drugs) to get well. Yet, we still despise natural means of healing but these will drive allopathic medical science to the wall and the day will come when its teachers will no longer be looked upon with scorn."

Tuberculin

We have all had experience how medical science daily seeks for new remedies to apply, because the old are no longer effectual. Recollect the blind enthusiasm for *tuberculin inoculations* before a single patient was even apparently cured; such a spectacle the world has surely never seen before. At first each new medicament paralyses the vital powers, but in time the system grows so insensible to it as no longer to react. As new and more potent remedy is now required to paralyse the vitality further until finally the fermentation of foreign matter cannot be longer prevented by any means at all and destruction of life is the result. An illustration will render this plainer.

"Any one who is learning to smoke has to battle with his stomach until the latter grows insensible to the poisonous nicotine. At first the stomach is vigorous enough to defend itself successfully against this poison but very soon its strength is weakened and complete insensibelity to the poison is the consequence. We now require a stranger poison than before to produce the first effect on the stomach."

Dr. Lindlahr says—"Some years ago a disease similar to small pox broke out among the sheep in certain parts of Scotland. As a preventive the sheep were vaccinated. In the course of a few years it was noticed that a great many ewes were unable to nourish their lambs; with the discontinuance of vaccination this phenomenon disappeared. Do not these facts help to explain why over fifty percent of human mothers are now incapable of nursing their babies."

"Looking forward—at present the trend of Allopathic medicine is undoubtedly towards the serum, antitoxin and vaccine treatment practically all medical research tends that way. Every now and then the medical journals and the medical papers announce new serums and antitoxins which are claimed to cure or create immunity to certain disease. Suppose the research and practice of medicine continue along with these lines and are generally accepted, or the medical associations would have it, and forced upon the public by law what would be the result? Before a child reached the years of adolescence it would have had injected into its blood the vaccines, serums and antitoxins of small pox, hydrophobia, tetanus, cerebro-spinal meningitis, typhoid fever, yellow fever, scarlet fever, malaria, diphtheria, pneumonia, tuberculosis, plague, cholera, etc. etc."

"If Allopathy were to have its way the blood of the adult would be a mixture of dozens of filthy bacterial extracts, disease taints and destructive drug poisons. The tonsils and adenoids, the appendix vermiformis and probably a few other parts of the human anatomy would be extirpated in early youth under compulsion of the health departments."

"Never was humanity" says Dr. Lindlahr M. D., "cursed by a blacker superstition than this, that disease can be cured and health maintained by the absorption of virulent poisons. Rational therapeutics will always eliminate morbid matter, and not introduce it into the system."

The author would suggest to the Health Department and the medical faculty of Bombay to investigate carefully and find out whether there were as many cases of tuberculosis, cancer and diabetes in Bombay before the vaccination was made compulsory and before vaccine and serum therapies were introduced into this town as thereafter. Saccharin, aspirin, and all coal tar preparations seem to increase the number of cases of cancer and the frequent use of aerated waters, sulphate of magnesium and the smoking habit to increase the death rate from heart failure.

Dr. J. S. Kramer, Cincinnati Institute, stated that a number of children died at the city Hospital from the serum used, and not from cerebro-spinal meningitis, as was supposed. The mortality was 14 out of 15 dying at the hospital, and five children died in five minutes after an injection of the Flexner serum (Herald of Health June 1919).

If we touch fire knowingly or unknowingly it burns; our ignorance of natural laws never lessens our suffering for it when we violate them; so also if we take poisons we must suffer the consequences whether we take them ignorantly or on the advice of some one, an ignorant quack, an experienced Vaid or thriving doctor diplomaed by the authorities. The administering of poisons to diseased persons is neither natural nor scientific.

Just imagine what the human blood will be like in coming generations if this artificial contamination with all sorts of disease taints and drug poisons is forced upon the people. As one particular system is patronised by Governments the adherents of it are trying their best to suppress the other systems and to perpetuate their own by taking advantage of the help given by Governments. It is really Nature that cures disease; therefore our mode of treatment should be to aid Nature in her efforts to heal and not to thwart her progress by introducing poisons either in the stomach or in the blood.

CHAPTER III.

Human body, its structure and natural functions

Man's superiority

Man is the master-piece of all Nature's products. She has formed his body in such a way that if proper care is taken, he should be able to live at least a century hale and hearty and free from all diseases. The peculiar structure of his brain with its wonderful power and the admirable mechanism of his hands with their different adaptations suitable to all the various purposes of worldly affairs have given him the superiority over the rest of the animal creation.

Human Body Compared to an Engine:— "The human body has been likened to a locomotive steam Engine with some important differences; there are striking analogies between these structures. In the one case there is food in the other coal. In the one case there is an incessant and considerable consumption of material which has become part and parcel of the various bodily organs; in the other the losses of the structure of mechanism itself are neither essential nor large. In both structures however carbon and hydrogen are burnt, yielding the same products. In both water is heated and vaporised; in both stored up or potential energy is converted into actual energy and heat. From both structures uncombustible or unused waste is thrown out." (*Prof. A. H. Church M. A.*).

Human body compared to a factory

"The human body may well be compared to a factory or work-shop, in the sense that the food represents the fuel, the mouth and gullet, the furnace, the stomach, the body of the furnace, the kidneys and liver, the ash grating and the bowels the ashpit. The lungs may be compared to the flues, the heat is the pulsometer and the nerves represent the electrical means of communication between the rooms of the factory" (Platen).

In the human body and in the locomotive, the fuel, is burned by the aid of air, the oxygen of which unites with the combustible part of the fuel, and the potential energy it contains is transformed into heat and power. The power of energy is used for muscular work the heat is used to keep up the body warm (Carrington).

Bodily Heat

" We cannot raise the temperature of animals above the normal standard by increasing the supply of hydro-carbons in the food, nor can we arrest the production of heat by depriving animals of the so-called calorific principles." (Flint M. D.)

Neither can we increase the temperature by making a person sit in the sun nor near the fire; nor can we decrease it by pouring cold water over him.

"We know that an electric current heats a wire along which it travels to do work and I suggest that, by analogy, *the vital energy* heats the body in following through it (the nervous mechanism) to do the mental and physical work of the organism—the work of the world. At least I can see no vital objection to this hypothesis (Carrington). Proof that the temperature is dependent upon the degree of vitality and not upon the extent of the food combustion is furnished by numerous observations of the phenomena of fasting (Carrington). When the body is clogged by over-eating, the production of heat is impeded. I am often asked " what food gives warmth and heat ? *No food does this.* Food may stimulate and produce sensations of warmth, but the body only is the heat producer." (Dr. Broadbent).

"There is no doubt that the oxygination of the tissues throughout the system and the combinations of oxygen with the carbon, are sources of animal heat, in common with all the organic functions and chemical changes which take place in the body. All the conditions requisite to the due regulation of the animal temperature, are good digestion, free respiration, vigorous circulation, proper assimilation, and perfect depuration, in two words.—*Good health*" (Carrington)

Human Life compared to a lamp.—Human Life may be compared to a lamp having a wick that would last a century. Both have heat (human heat being 98·6 on the thermometer). Both require a supply of fresh atmosphere. Man requires food with oily ingredients ; the lamp requires a wick containing oil. In both there is consumption of material. In both oxygen is required ; in both carbon is burnt. Both can produce species of their own. If proper care is not taken and if improper food is supplied, man is exposed to disease which may terminate in premature death. If exposed to rough wind butterflies, dust, etc.—and if dirty oil is used the ordinary life of the lamp may be cut short.

Changes and wastes that occur in the body

The human body consists of fluids and solids constantly changing from one into other, from the moment of its inception—a continual change of elements takes place in the different organs and its size, weight, strength and the quantity of its fluids and solids differ according to age. In youth the fluids are more than in old age. Such changes are natural and necessary to life.

Loss and Gain in Human Body.—A man neither loses nor gains weight when he eats just enough to make up for the waste.

A child assimilates more than what it loses and is thus gaining weight and increases in size—while an old man eats less and assimilates less than what he loses and thus loses weight and strength day by day.

The average daily loss and supply caused in the body—The quantity of waste matter daily thrown off by the body in the form of perspiration is carbonic acid water in different forms and the solid excrements, amounts to nearly one-twentieth part of persons entire weight. Thus a man weighing 160 lbs will throw off daily, if in health, about 8 lbs of waste matter, and in order to balance this loss he needs about 8 lbs. of food. (J. Ernst M. D.)

The Structure of Human body—Its organs and their Natural Functions.—The human body is separable into the head, trunk, and limbs, the skeleton includes the bones of the whole of the human frame.

The skull is formed of twenty-two bones, eight of which compose the cranium and fourteen the face. These form cavities for the organs of senses, viz.

(1) The eyes for seeing,
(2) The ears for hearing,
(3) The nose for smelling and breathing,
(4) The mouth for eating, talking, &c.

The trunk consists of the chest and the abdomen and supports the head.

The limbs are attached to the trunk and are connected to the head internally by the nervous system and are at the command as it were of the brain.

The chest is situated between the neck and the abdomen and contains the heart, lungs and large blood vessels.

The other organs may be grouped into the following systems.

(1) The Nervous system
(2) The Circulatory System
(3) The Respiratory System
(4) The Digestive System
(5) The Excretory System
A.—Urinary System
B.—Cutaneous System
(6) The reproductory generative system.

(1) *The nervous system* :—comprises the brain, spinal cord, nerves, and ganglia (groups of nerve cells or the

sympathetic system.) The brain is enclosed in the cavity of the skull and is protected by three fibrous membranes (coverings) called the meninges.

The cerebrum or large brain lies upper most and the cerebellum or small brain is behind and below the former. There are numerous layers of nerve cells in the brain and they are furnished nutrition by the numerous blood and lymph vessels.

Olfactory, auditory, gustatory and other nerves of special sense arise in the brain which is the centre of all the senses and serve as telegraph-wires and serve the purpose of carrying messages (sensation) to and from the brain are in the blood they are proteids, salts of various kinds, oil, sugar, etc.—various tissue wastes which are to be exerted in the form of perspiration are also found in it.

A large bundle of nerves proceeding from the right side of the brain down to the spinal column crosses over the left side in the spinal cord and *vice versa*, and this is the reason why an injury to the brain causes paralysis of the opposite side of the body. Motor nerves carry messages from the brain to the muscles and sensory nerves carry the sensations of touch, pain, etc to the brain; solar-plexus, a ganglia which is the centre of vitality is situated just above the pit of the stomach and sympathises with the heart and the stomach. The lumbar ganglia attends to the intestines. The nerves of the liver, the spleen and the kidneys, the intestines and all the visceral organs belong to the sympathetic system.

(2) *The circulatary system* :—

Importance of the blood :—By incessant vital work which continues even during sleep the molecular elements of the organism are wasted and have to be replaced by new ones. This important work is done by the blood. The food supplies the blood the necessaries and thus serves indirectly to repair the waste of the body.

"The blood is the medium through which nourishment is conveyed to all parts of the body and it serves at the same time to wash out all the waste effete matters from the tissues and organs." (Dr. Hehir).

The blood in the body weighs one thirteenth part of it. It contains 40 per cent of little bodies called cells. All the elements required for building and repair of the body are in the blood. They are proteids, salts of various kinds, oil, sugar, etc.; various tissue wastes which are to be excreted in the form of perspiration are also found in it.

The heart is situated in the cavity of the chest and is the centre of the circulatory system. It weighs eight to ten ounces and lies on the left side, only one third of it being on the right side of the middle line of the body. It is enclosed in an envelope called pericardium and is lined into a thin and fibrous membrane which is termed endocardium.

The valves of the heart are of fibrous membranes so placed as to allow the stream of the blood to flow in one direction only. This is Nature's arrangement to keep the bood always circulating through the body.

Blood vessels are of three varieties, viz. arteries, nerves and capillaries. The arteries are vessels composed of muscles, connectives and elastic tissues that carry the blood from the heart, while the veins are thin and less elastic and carry the blood to the heart. Capillaries are numerous thin small vessels which are distributed all over the body and are so small as to require the aid of a microscope to see them.

Process of circulation.

The blood is driven from the left side of the heart through the arteries over the body into the capillaries and is collected in the veins and thence carried to the right side of the heart from which it passes through the lungs.

The lungs are the organs which purify the blood in the system by absorbing the oxygen of the inhaled air.

(3) *The respiratory system* :—The lungs are the respiratory organs, they are two in number and occupy the greater part of the cavity of the thorax and partially cover the heart. The air inhaled through the nose enters the larynx or voice organ, the trachea, the wind pipe and the bronchial tubes. Bronchial tubes are two in number one going to each lung.

The right lung is divided into three lobes and the left into two. Each lung is covered with a delicate membrane called pleura.

The lungs consist of numerous minute sacs or air-cells with small tubes opening into them; the tubes are covered and surrounded with blood vessels.

These blood vessels break up into capillaries and carry the impure venous blood which comes into contact with the air inhaled and replenished with oxygen. Here the air in the aircells of the lung loses oxygen and gets loaded with carbonic acid.

In the process of respiration the inhaled air thus loses five per cent of oxygen and gains the same amount of carbonic acid as much watery vapour as it can hold and certain quantity of decaying animal matter. Hence the necessity of breathing pure air.

Pure air is absolutely essential both to the sick and healthy in all diseases, at all times and under all circumstances. It is the pure air that sustains our life. We can live for a few weeks without food for few days without water but we cannot live even for a few minutes without air.

(4) *The digestive system* :—includes the mouth, the salivary glands, the pharynx, the aesophagus, the stomach, the liver, the pancreas (sweet bread) and the intestines.

When food is being masticated in the mouth the saliva from the salivary glands mixes with it and aids digestion. It is then conveyed down the œsophagus or gullet through pharynx and passed into the stomach.

The pharynx is the upper part of the œsophagus, a muscular bag at the back of the mouth receiving the food and conveying it to the stomach. The œsophagus is lined with mucous membrane and is about nine inches long. The stomach is an elongated bag capable of holding about 40 to 45 ounces of liquid.

The mucous membrane of the stomach contains numerous small glands resembling tubes which secrete a fluid called the gastric juice. The portions of the food already dissolved are absorbed into the system through the stomach walls.

The liver is the largest gland in the body and is situated below the ribs on the right side. It secretes the bile which prevents the decomposition of the food in the intestines and turns it to the best possible use of the body.

Pancreas or sweet bread secretes a fluid called pancreatic juice. The bile is stored up in the gall-bladder. The bile duct is joined by the duct from the pancreas and thus bile and pancreatic fluid are conveyed into the duodenum. Duodenum is the first part of the small intestine. The food thus passes on into the small and thence into the large intestines. "The interior of the intestines is lined by the mucous membrane containing glands of various kinds in the different regions" (Dr. Humphry). While the food thus passes through the walls of the small and large intestines the process of absorption is continued and the further the food progresses within the intestines the more are its liquid portions drawn off till what is left is only an indegestible remainder which is ultimately excreted through the anus. (Ernst M. D.)

(5) *The Excretory System* :—

(A) *Urinary* system—" The excretory system comprises the glands and their excretory parts by means of which the blood is enabled to get rid of the waste products. The kidneys are the largest and most important of the excretory glands. They are two in number, of dark-purple colour and in shape like a french bean. They are situated in the loins at the back of the abdominal cavity, one on either side of the lumbar vertabrae of the spine. A duct called the ureter passes down from each kidney and opens into the bladder. The bladder forms a bag which lies in the pelvis in the lower abdomen. The urine is secreted by the kidneys, is passed down the ureters, and is collected in the bladder, being got rid of from time to time through the urinary passage (Dr. Humphry).

(B) *Cutaneous systeem;*—

The skin not only acts as a covering to the body, but it is also an organ of excretion and contains glands which serve this purpose namely the sweat glands and the sebaceous glands; water and sundry impurities are extracted from the blood and poured on to the surface of the skin in the form of sweat by the sweat glands. The sebaceous glands supply a fatty or oily fluid which lubricates the skin. Nails and hair are modifications of the superficial layer of the skin (Dr. Humphry).

The covering skin is called the epidermis while the inner lining (skin) is called the dermis. The outer skin is formed of many layers of cells; it is also called cuticle or scar skin. It is a protection to the more sensitive inner skin which consists of a fine but strong network of connective tissue. The deeper part of the inner skin is connected to the tissues under the skin such as muscle or bone by a very loose connective tissue of varying thickness called subcutaneous tissue. It (dermis) is also supplied with blood-vessels.

The Skin

(1) The skin is a medium for purification of the blood and protection of the bodies.

(2) It extracts from our food what is needed through mucous membrane to repair the waste in the flesh.

(3) It extracts from the light, air and water certain energies needed for our bodies.

(4) It conveys the nervous impulses to the brain through the nerves.

(5) It assists our lungs in respiration.

(6) It assists our kidneys in excretion.

The skin is not only an important secretory organ, besides the lungs, intestines and kidneys but also a respiratory organ and an apparatus for controlling our internal warmth. It is a faithful mirror of our internal conditions as it has intimate relations with the function of every single organ in the body. The state of our skin reacts on the welfare or disease of our entire organism and this in its turn reacts on the health of the outer skin (Platen).

"The skin is the great heat regulator of the body... The net work of the circulation in the skin is said to be so capacious that it could contain one half to two-thirds of the total circulating blood.

The more active this circulation and the more blood present in the skin, the higher is its temperature and the greater the loss of bodily heat. When on the other hand the circulation in the skin is contracted, its temperature falls and the loss of heat is deminished (Dr. Fox M. D. Lond).

The skin is a great absorber of energy, as every one who has been exposed to the solar rays must have experienced. This nervous surface organ is constantly engaged in receiving and transmitting to the centres in the brain and spinal cord an infinite number of impressions from the outside world (Dr. Fox M.D.Lond).

"The skin is a vast secretary and excretary glandular organ. The amount of the daily perspiration of an adult in an atmosphere at 100° F. is estimated at 30 oz. as compared wlth 15 oz of water thrown off by the lungs. It is said that the pressure of the perspiration in the sweat-gland exeeds that in the large arteries. A considarable amount of carbonic acid gas is contained in the sweat estimated at about one thirtieth of that exhaled from the lungs. The nitrogenous, matter, urea, etc., excreted by the skin may amount to 4 or 5 percents of that contained in the urine. It is interesting to note that when the function of the kidneys fails a compensating power of the skin comes into play and the cutaneous excretion of nitrogenous waste may be greatly increased. (Dr. Fox M. D. Lond).

We have on us an outer skin
Another skin we have within.
The inner is a lining in

All over as a membrane thin;
That cuticle which we see out
Is doubled and led in throughout.
Mouth, palate, windpipe, nose and throat
All are lined with this inner coat
From mouth to anus, end to end
Through every part it doth extend
The inner skin extracts from food
All what is needed for our good
While outer one exudes from flesh
What we don't need and doth refresh
Our bodies in a mystic way
And doth keep all disease away
It doth extract from atmosphere
Pure oxygen; it is its sphere.
It takes from water, air and light
Some energy and keeps us bright.
It aids lungs in inhaling air
And thus helps them health to repair
Exuding dregs from body too
It renders kidneys its help due.
It doth convey through all our nerves
An impulse to the brains and serves
As guardian and sentinel
Of life, and does its duty well.
If much dirt we accumulate
On the skin or it suffocate
By not allowing fresh pure air
To touch it, how can it repair
Our body and mind to sound state ?

And how can it waste compensate ?
So long skin outer is quite well
Through it our blood dregs will expel
If anything goes wrong with blood
Our skin will soon nip it in bud
And suffer itself for blood's sake
And its own good health it will stake
Hence we should always promptly take
Great care of skin which doth partake
All sufferings of inner flesh
And blood, and tries them to refresh
If we take its care properly
It will serve for a century
And will keep us free from disease
By giving comfort, peace and ease.
  But we don't daily wash it well
And thus it can not dregs expel
Nor we allow it to inhale
Pure air there-by we don't get hale
We suffocate it day and night
By wearing thick clothes close and tight
Apply scents and worst scented soap
And dont allow it to have scope
To do its functions easily
And to impart us health and glee.
If it tries its best to relieve
Blood from ills, that we dont believe
Instead of thanking for what's done
We do try to have it undone
By external drugs poisonous
Thereby we do great harm to us

We thus live with disease and fears
For less than three scores and ten years
If natural food we partake
And use of Nature's gifts we make
And proper care of skin we take
Both day and night for our health's sake
We can live over hundred years
Quite free from all disease and tears.

Nails :—

A nail consists of epidermis and is formed by the outer corneous cells to which it owes its hardness. Though the growth of the nails is the same both in health and during illness, the portion of the nail formed during the progress of debilitating diseases will be perceptibly thinner than that produced during health.

Hair :—

A hair is composed of horny cells and is formed from the epidermis. It lies in a deep pit called the hair follicle from the bottom of which it springs. It is a bad conductor of heat and electricity.

Purpose of the hair :—It is supplied by Nature both as an ornament to the head and as a protection to the brain and eye sight from the effects of the sun and excessive heat in summer, of extreme cold in winter and of lightning in rainy season.

Eyebrows :—

The eyebrows and eyelids are beautifully adopted for the defence of the organs of vision. The small hairs which grow in the apertures of the nostrils serve as guardians to the delicate membrane of the nose. Being situated in the entrance of the lungs they promote warmth to the air inhaled and are intended to afford protection from injurious effects of rapid variations of the atmosphere and give immunity from the diseases of the respiratory system if breathing is practised through the nostrils and not through mouth.

Moustache and beard.

Moustache and beard :—not only impart manly grace to the human face but also serve as protection to all the glands in the mouth and throat and the whole of the respiratory system.

"There can be no doubt" says Mr Chadwick that the moustache is a natural respirator defending the lungs against the inhalation of dust and cold; it is a defence of the throat and face against the cold and it is equally in warm climates a protector of those parts against excessive heat." It also would be of services to labourers in all dusty trades and to travellers on dusty roads. Persons who rear moustaches and beard are less susceptible to tooth-ache than others who are void of them; and their teeth also are less apt to decay. Those who keep beard are immune from the attacks of mumps, tonsillitis, sore throat, bronchitis and other inflammatory diseases of the respiratory organs.

Every hair on the surface of the human body supplied by Nature is for the purpose of protecting that part on which its grows. It is also intended by her to drive out certain impurities from the body as it separates a large quantity of carbon and hydrogen from the system.

6. *Generative System; Progeny at will :—*

Two separate germs are required for the reproduction of the human species; one is the ovum which is developed in the ovaries of women and the other spermatozoon which is developed in the testicles of men; when these two meet in the action of sexual intercourse the embroy begins to develop in the womb.

The ovum of the female element in reproduction is a cell with a smaller nucleus in the larger one (the neucleolus) and a well-defined cell membrane (zona-pellucida) Around it are numerous cells clinging to it from which it probably draws nourishment (the discus prolegerus) (Barclay).

The spermatozoon is a modified cell. The original cell lengthens out into a vibratile tail (compare the flagella of heteromita) which gives it power of movement. While the nucleus advances in the opposite direction towards the head. (Barclay).

Dr. Sext, a German physician has discovered that the right testicle of man and the right ovary of woman respectively produced sperm and germ capable of producing a male child and those of the left testicle and left ovary capable of producing a femele child. He also found out that no conception can take place by the conjunction of the sperm of the right testicle with the germ of the left ovary or by conjunction of the sperm of the left testicle with the germ of the right ovary.

Dr. Trall, an American physician verified the truth of Dr. Sext's discovery by experimenting on some animals. He castrated the right testicle of a dog and kept him with a bitch and she bore only female young ones. But that very bitch produced some male and some female pups when she was kept with another dog having both testicles. He then castrated the left ovary of that bitch and kept her again with the dog whose right testicle was castrated, there was no issue at all; but when she was kept with another dog whose left testicle was castrated she produced only male young ones. So also when a dog whose left testicle was castrated was allowed to live with several bitches and they all produced male pups only; while a dog whose right testicle was castrated was allowed to live with several bitches they all gave birth to female young ones. Several experiments of this nature were made by Dr. Trall on dogs, cats and other animals with the results of the same nature which went to verify the statement of Dr. Sext.

Dr. Trall also states that, at the time of sexual intercourse, one of the testicles rises slightly higher than the other, it is a sign that the semen from that testicle is being ejaculated then. From this he concludes that if a man raises his right testicle either at the time of commencing sexual intercourse or in the course of it there will be every probability of getting a male child provided conception takes place then. In the same way if the left testicle is raised there will be a probability of having a female offspring. He says the testi[illegible] may be mechanically raised by means of a finger or by the use of a thin soft cloth strap tied to the waist. He also states that several of his friends were able to produce progeny at their will at his suggestion by observing the above method.

Nature's sole object of sexual intercourse is the propagation of one's own species. The act is enjoined with pleasurable emotion by Her as the parties should not shirk from their proper duties. Primitive human beings obeyed Her command strictly in this affair. But the human beings of present day have become the victims of morbid abnormal desire and morbid actions. Unnatural heat-producing food, stimulating and intoxicating drinks, the use of narcotics, late hours, etc. cause undue abnormal desire. Unnatural social customs, false modesty, bad economy make them devise unnatural methods of gratification. The preservation of species is not taken into consideration at all. On the contrary some are not only displeased but are annoyed by the fact that this action fulfils Nature's purpose which they are trying to frustrate, and thus devise so many unnatural measures against Nature's process for which they cannot escape unpunished. They should all remember well that Nature is a strict sentinel and she chastises all the defaulters.

CHAPTER IV.

Human Life and its natural wants.

Human life has been already compared to a lamp; every one is aware that if proper care is not taken man is subject to disease and premature death. He has some natural appetites and they must be satisfied according to Nature's laws. They are :—

1 Breathing, 2 Thirst, 3 Hunger 4 Sleep and 5 Sexual gratification. The first four wants tend to sustain his own life and the last one to maintain his health and to propagate his species.

1 Breathing

Breathe always through the nostrils and not through the mouth. Breathing is divided into two respiratory actions, (1) Inspiration by which the lungs are expanded and the air is drawn in and down in the wind-pipe; and (2) expiration by which the lungs are contracted and the air is forced out of the wind-pipe.

Pure air contains

Oxygen	21
Nitrogen	78
Carbonic acid	0·033
Watery vapour, ammonia, traces of organic and inorganic substances	0·967
Total	100·000

The expired air differs from inspired or pure atmospheric air in the following points.

(1) The expired air becomes nearly as hot as the blood.

(2) It is charged with more watery matter.
(3) It loses five percent of its oxygen.
(4) It gains five percent of carbonic acid.
(5) It gains a great quantity of decaying animal matter.

This considerable reduction of oxygen and addition of carbonic acid and decaying animal matter renders air impure and it becomes injurious to those who inhale it. To preserve the natural heat of the body and to render the blood pure in the region of the heart during the course of its circulation a pure supply of oxygen through inhaled air is indispensable. Hence the necessity of living in fresh and pure atmosphere.

2 Thirst.

Absence of thirst with a continuous flow of saliva in the mouth is a sign of good health. The use of salt, chillies, condiments, sugar, tobacco, alcohol, etc. will cause thirst in healthy persons.

In all inflammatory diseases, chiefly fevers, there is abnormal thirst. In diabetes mellitus and insipidus also the patient has inclination to drink frequently. Pickles, jams, fried things, and other heaty food may also cause abnormal thirst. In summer when the skin perspires more freely even healthy persons are likely to get abnormal thirst.

In such cases the natural and most agreeable mode of quenching it is to eat a juicy fruit or drink water from a tender cocoanut; chewing a piece of sugarcane and drinking the juice of it is also an excellent mode of quenching thirst. If these things are not available a little pure cold water may be sipped frequently. Even in fevers it is a most soothing beverage; a little fruit juice may be added to it whenever convenient.

Tea, coffee, aerated waters, beer, wine, syrup, etc. are not suitable for quenching thirst. They are all drugs diluted in water and will not suit the purpose of quenching thirst. (For full details see Scientific Hydropathy by the author).

3 Hunger

Eat only when you are hungry. Make it a habit to eat at regular intervals and eat only the substances intended by Nature for human consumption. Masticate your food well and ivsalivate it properly before you swallow it.

Dr. Page says—"In accordance with a universal law of Nature the conservation of energy, gastric juice, upon which digestion depends, is secreted from the blood by the glands of the stomach in proportion to the needs of the organism for food, and not in proportion to the amount of food swallowed. There is therefore a normal dyspepsia for whatever of excess is taken. Moreover in such cases, none of the food is well digested."

Nutrition solely and and wholely depends on the power of digestion and assimilation. It is not the food consumed but the food assimilated that affords nutrition. Material is different in different kinds of food. Food fired, heated, boiled, baked, cooked, fried, salted, sugared, spiced, pickled, preserved, etc. loses its nutritive value partly or entirely and according to the harmful substances added to it and the artificial process to which it is subjected. All these substances are not natural and are sure to impede digestion and do some harm to the digestive organs. Only fresh fruits, nuts, cereals, etc. which can be eaten fresh without any artificial interference if properly masticated and insalivated are properly digested and they supply proper nutrition and tend to preserve health and energy.

Those food-stuffs which are disgusting to sight and smell in their crude form and are cooked and seasoned before eating are most injurious to health, however tasty they may become after being seasoned. Fish, fowl and fleshmeat come under this class of food.

Those food-stuffs which are not repulsive to sight, not disgusting to smell, not distasteful to the tongue and which can be easily masticated by our teeth and easily swallowed by the throat with pleasure and without any difficulty after being insalivated are easily digested by the stomach and are good for our health. Fruits, nuts, sugarcanes, berries, green and fresh tender vegetable come under this classs of food.

Prof. Chittendon says :—

" The so called cravings of appetite are purely the result of habit. A habit once acquired and persistently followed soon has us in its grasp, and then any deviation there-from disturbs our physiological equilibrium. The sytem makes complaint and we experience a craving, it may be, for that to which the body has been accustomed, even though this something be, in the long run distinctly injurious to the welfare of the body

There has thus come about a sentiment that the cravings or the appetite for food are to be fully satisfied, and this is merely obedience to Nature's laws. The idea is however fundamentally wrong. Anyone with a little persistence can change his or her habits of life, change the whole order of cravings thus demonstrating that the latter are purely artificial and that they have no necessary connection with the welfare or needs of the body. In other words, dietatic requirements are to be founded not upon so called instinct and craving but upon reason and intelligence."

"A great many are dying slowly from auto-intoxication, food poisoning, wrong habits, over eating and under breathing. Many people today are eating too much and hurrying themselves to the grave. It is time that some simple truths were taught in the public schools about the care of the human body. Every child should be taught first how to preserve health and attain a ripe old age, and the knowledge afterwards gained would be of some benefit; whereas at the present time we find our children on the verge of nervous prostration before they gradute and many die before the prime of life. Over 90 per cent of disease is caused by error in diet, eating too much food, too larg a quantity of either the proteids, fats or carbohydrates or wrong combinations of food". (Carrington).

Natural food-stuffs, their constituents and their use.

Almonds contain oil, proteids and phosphorus, and are useful as a general tonic both to the body and brains.

Apples contain phosphates of calcium, potash and soda, albumen, chlorophyle, malic acid, lime, gum, sugar, etc., and they cure acidity, dyspepsia, colic, diarrhoea, disorders of liver and kidneys, such as gall-stones, and renal calculi. They are very useful for general debility.

Asparagus contains potash, phosphates of potash and soda. It is a diuretic and is useful for scanty urine palpitation of the heart and worm troubles.

Bananas or plantains contain phosperus, iron, soda, albumen, starch, etc. The red contain more of iron and sugar and are good for anaemia and general debility; the yellow contain more of soda and are useful for constipation; the green contain more of potash and soda and are diuretic.

Barley contains starch, gluten, albumen, oil, salts and hordeic acid. It is laxative diuretic and tonic.

Cabbage contains sulphur, soda and iron; it is useful for coughs, bronchitis, asthma, warts and some skin diseases.

Capsicum or chilli is a pungent stimulating medicine and not a daily food-stuff. It increases the secretion of saliva, gastric juice and every sort of liquid substance in the body just to have an after-effect or reaction. It causes burning in many parts of the body and great thirst later on. It contains iron, soda, and some acids; it is useful for chills, fever accompanied with chills, flatulence, stomach pains, rheumatism, etc.; it can stop toothache also temporarily if its tincture is applied to the seat of pain.

Carrot :—contains silicea, calicium and sodium salts and is useful for gouty patients as it eliminates uric acid from the system; it also prevents brick-dust-like sediments in the urine. It brings the liver in proper order and cures gall-stone troubles also.

Celery :—contains iron and sulphur and is good for rheumatism and gout.

Cherry :—contains sodium salts and is useful for urinary troubles.

Chest nut :—contains fluorine, calcium, kalium and ferrum salts and is useful for blind piles, pain in waist, hernia, congestion of liver, etc.

Cinnamon is a medicine and not a food stuff. It contains tannin, cinnamic acid, resin, sugar, and traces of potash. It is a remedy for flatulence, cancer, and haemorrhages of black blood.

Clove:—is also a medicine and not a food stuff. If moderately taken it cures dyspepsia; but in large quantities it has an opposite action. Externally it is useful for toothache and also for neuralgic and rheumatic pains.

Cocoanut :—contains phosphates of calcium, iron, potash and soda; it contains also milky and oily substance, albumen and a little starch. It is a valuable substitute for milk, ghee, codliver oil, and all its preparations. It is very easily assimilated; more easily than milk and codliver oil; the weak and the tubercular patients can safely make use of it both as food and general tonic. It is more strengthening than soups.

Currents :—contain iron, sodium and sugar; black ones contain more of iron than other sorts; they are cooling and laxative and are useful for constipation, scanty urine, fever and anaemia.

Custard-apple :—contains soda, potash, sulphur and sugar. It is cooling and refreshing; it cures obstinate boils and carbuncles; the pulp prepared from its leaves can cure them sooner than surgeon's knife and doctor's poisonous mixtures.

Dates :—Contain 20 percent of pure sugar and some valuable phosphates, chiefly of iron. They prevent constipation and soothe the heart. They must be eaten with grated cocoanut as they are otherwise too sweet for the taste and are very heaty.

Figs :—are laxative, they contain sugar, phosphates, gum, albumen, etc.

Flax or linseed contains acetic acid, acetate and muriate of potash. It is useful for congestion, inflamation, cough, etc. It promotes expectration in coughs, consumption, tuberculosis, and is useful for hectic fever, night sweats, urinary difficulties, etc. One ounce of linseed, half an ounce of liquorice roots must be mixed in a pound of water and reduced to 8 ounces by boiling and taken with a few drops of lemon juice and a little honey. It is called linseed tea.

Garlic is a great disinfectant; it contains some strong odoured acid. It cures obstinate sores and tuberculosis. Small pieces of garlic should be eaten with grated cocoanut and lemon juice. It can be used externally also.

Gooseberies:—contain citric acid, chloride of potash and sodium, gum, sugar, water and albumen. They are good for biliousness, constipation and dyspepsia.

Grapes—are rich in sugar called glucose; they contain tannin, gum, tartrate of lime, magnesia, alum, iron, chloride of potash and soda, tartaric, citric and malic acid, etc. The rind or skin of grapes is astringent and constipating and the juice and pulp are laxative and they allay thirst and are useful for that reason in fevers and hot seasons. They are useful for children during teething and whenever they are constipated They promote flow of urine and are useful in gout and rheumatism. Cancer patients will do well by eating a large quantity of them.

Hazel nuts contain sulphur, oil, protein, etc., and are useful for bleeding piles, haematuria and haemorrhages of dark blood from any orifice.

Honey contains glucose or grape sugar, phosphates, and some aromatics. It is the best substitute for sugar, jam, jelly, etc. and is useful in coughs, consumption of lungs, dyspepsia and also for boils and carbuncles.

Jackfruit is rich in sugar, albumen and calcium and soda salts. It is yellow inside when ripe and is laxative. Dyspetics should not venture to eat it in a large quantity as it is difficult to digest.

Jambools contain sodium salts and sugar and are useful for diabetes mellitus and diarrhoea.

Kajunuts contain soda, iron, and traces of silicea; both fruits and nuts are very heaty. The best time to eat the nuts is when they are tender.

Lemon contains potassium chloride, citrate, malate, and tartaric acid; therefore it serves as an antibilious and antiscorbutic. It is also rich in vitamines. It cures spongy gums, scurvy, biliousness, dyspepsia, gout, rheumatism, constipation, sore throat, thirst, heart burn, lumbago and coughs simple or phthisical. It is also useful for liver and spleen troubles and may prevent malarial fever if continued long. It is also good for obesity and muco-colitis of long standing.

Lettuce—contains potassium salts and is useful for sleeplessness.

Liquorice :—contains sugar, iron, sodium, etc. and is useful for coughs, and inflammatory conditions; it is a household remedy for coughs with linseed and lemon-juice and for dry cough, bronchitis, asthma, pneumonia, etc. and also for boils, carbuncles, etc.

Maize contains calcium, iron and soda salts and starch which is easily turned into sugar. It is as strengthening as wheat though it contains less starch and more salts. It can be eaten with grated cocoanut.

Mangoes contain sugar and highly refined turpentine in them ; they also contain iron, useful acid and they are useful for rheumatism, diarrhoea, diabetes, etc. Their seeds and rinds are astringent.

Milk serves both as food and drink. When fresh milk is not available a cup of milk may be kept in boiling water for about 15 or 20 minutes and when it becomes tepid may be taken with or without fruit juice but without sugar. Milk is an excellent ingredient to quench thirst during illness, fatigue and in hot weather.

Millet contains soda, lime and iron salts, etc., it is nutritious and laxative; It can be chewed and eaten when it is in its juicy condition. Its breads may be eaten with grated cocoanut or any fruits.

Oats (*java*)—Contains sodium, potassium, calcium and kalium salts; it is a very nourishing food. It is useful for diabetic patients as it contains sodium salts and less of *starch than any other grain.*

Onions:—contain sulphur, phosphorus, potassium salts, ammonia, phosphoric and acetic acids, citrate of lime, starch, sugar, ligumine and volatile oil, etc; they are a household remedy for cough, bronchitis, scanty urine, colds, influenza, liver troubles, inflammatory conditions, gout, rheumatism, etc. they promote perspiration and circulation of blood.

Oranges:—Contain citric acid, citrate of potash, albumen, sugar, water, sodium and iron. In influenza, plague and dengue if they are eaten freely, they will prevent pneumonia and other troubles. It is a good remedy for dyspepsia, asthma, liver troubles, coughs, bronchitis, heart troubles, typhoid fever, etc.

Papaya (carica) cantains sodium and calcium salts and is useful for dyspepsia, liver and spleen troubles; but is very heaty. Pregnant women should not venture to eat a large quantity of it.

Peach contains iron, gum, sugar and acids. It is a tonic and aperient and is useful for fever, and anæmia.

Pears contain nitric acid, pectose, gums, sugar, albumen and some valuable salts. Its external skin or rind is laxative *but the inner* portion has the property of constipating the bowels. It is a very pleasant fruit. Its leaves can be made into an excellent tooth brush; they are better than all the tooth remedies in the market.

Peas and Beans :—contain starch, albumen, sulphur, potash and calcium salts. They cause flatulence and uric acid. In small quantities, if well masticated and insalivated properly, and digested, they are nutritive and strength-giving.

Pine-apple—Contains muriatic acid, a constituent of gastric juice and is useful for dyspepsia. It dissolves albumen and is a useful remedy in obesity, Bright's disease, diphtheria, etc.

Pomegranate contains sugar potash and sodium salts. It is an astringent food and is useful for diarrhoea, dysentery, sprue, worm troubles, etc. a strong decoction of its root-bark is an excellent remedy for tapeworm.

Plums and prunes contain potassium salts and sugar and are cooling and refreshing; they are gentle laxatives. They are useful in nervous deseases, irritability, dyspepsia, constipation, etc.

Potato contains citric acid, potash salts, phosphoric acid, starch and water. It is a very nutritious food. It can be used for poultices in indolent ulcers.

Radish is rich in soda and is a remedy for dyspepsia, piles, gall-stones, renal calculi, constipation, colic, etc.

Rice is rich in ferrum salts, starch, etc., and is a good food in diarrhoea, dysentery, fevers, etc. Its pericarp or bran is rich in sodium, potash and calcium salts and is a good remedy in constipation, dyspepsia, weakness and in some skin diseases.

Spinach:—contains ferrum salts. Some species contain ferrum and sodium salts and are good for dyspepsia, constipation, fever, urinary troubles, etc.

Straw berries:—are rich in citric acid and sodium salts and are laxative. They are useful in fever, rheumatism, gout, etc. The leaves and roots are astringent and are useful for diarrhoea and dysentery.

Sweet lime:—(*Musambi*) is an excellent food-stuff both during health and illness. It contains phosphates of calcium, iron, potash and soda. It also contains citric acid and citrate of potash; the fruit lasts even 3 or 4 weeks if properly preserved and is useful even in worst type of typhoid fever, smallpox, dengue, influenza, cholera, constipation, colic and worm troubles.

Tomatoes:—contain citric and malic acids and also calcium and soda salts; they also contain phosphates of iron, oxalate of potash and sugar and are suited to anaemic and bilious patients but not to gouty persons.

Turnip contains sulphur, potassium and sodium salts; so it is an aperient and diuretic.

Walnuts—contain phosphorus, phosphates of potash, calcium and magnesium and are suited to brain workers and persons of weak constitution; but they must be eaten very sparingly as they are very heaty and cause constipation; walnut oil is a remedy for eczema and other obstinate skin diseases. The tincture prepared from its rind cures obstinate eczema if taken in Homeopathic doses. Its unripe fruits are useful for worm troubles and the decoction prepared from its leaves (1 oz. to 10 oz of water) is a cure for sore throat, scrofulous ulcers, indolent sores, etc. One ounce of decoction is taken thrice a day. It is also used to wash obstinate and chronic sores.

Water-melon contains iron potassium and sodium and also a large quantity of sugar and water. It is an excellent fruit to quench thirst.

Wheat—contains all the nutritive biochemic salts and phosphates required for the subsistence of human body; calcium, iron, potash, and soda salts, water, fat, starch, albumen, etc. which are required for the human body are in wheat; so it may be styled as a perfect food for human consumption.

Man can sustain only on wheat for months and even years. Wheat among the cereals, milk among the animal food stuffs, plantains among fruits and cocoanuts among nuts can be styled as perfect foods for human consumption. One can sustain on each of these for years without any other food and without losing energy.

4 Sleep

Do not sleep during day time.

Do not keep up late at night.

Keep open all the windows of your sleeping compartment.

"Airy, well-ventilated, sleeping apartments" says Dr. Ruddock " should be ranked as the most important requirement of life both in health and disease." Sleep in the open air or in a room where there is ample provision of fresh air will be more refreshing and invigorating than in a room where fresh air is not freely admitted. "The air of an apartment," he adds, "containing several human beings, if unchanged, not only becomes charged with carbonic acid gas, but also gets impregnated with animal particles which fly off from the skin and lungs and are so minute as scarcely to be detected by the microscope but capable of decomposition and which taken by the breath into the lungs, may be absorbed and may develop the worst forms of diseases."

If you suffer from sleeplessness do not take bromide of potassium, morphia, opium or chloral hydrate. They do not produce healthy sleep but they cause stupor and the patient gets up in the morning with exhausted feeling. A hot foot-both is an effective measure for inducing natural and refreshing sleep.

5 Sexual Gratification

For sexual gratification wed a person whom you love and who loves you ardently in return. It is not the most beautiful person that gives you pleasure and happiness but the person who loves you heartily; besides you cannot expect to have a healthy and intelligent child from a person who does not love you in return. Further, such a person cannot supply proper animal magnetism to you and compensate for the loss sustained by the intercourse. Loveless marriages and mercenary intercourse will do greater harm than abstinence. Long abstinence also does some harm to the general health than excess. Starvation impedes digestive power more than over-eating; the same rule holds good in sexual appetite also.

Marriages with the nearest blood relations chiefly with cousins are very objectionable. They either extinguish love or bring forth no children. And if children be born they are weak in intellect and physique. Either of the couple as well as their children very often die prematurely. There are instances of families becoming extinct by reason of such marriages taking place continuously for some generations. The immutable Law of Nature is:

Two similar things must repel
Each other as if like a spell
While things dissimilar attract
Each other always in their act.

This universe is full of beautiful things; how beautiful is the rising sun? How attractive is the midday sun with his scorching rays? How tempting is the setting sun with his golden rays? How charming are the lotuses in ponds? Peacock, deer and other animals, trees and creepers with different coloured fragrant flowers and fruits really present a most alluring scene. How beautiful is the canopy of heaven with its starry vault and the moon presenting different phases on different days? The celebrated Sanskrit poet Kalidas says that the moon is so beautiful, the dark spots on her instead of marring her charms have made her look more charming. The roaring sea, the running streams, and rivers, the high majestic mountains and dark clouds with dazzling lightning are all attractive to the human eye.

But to a healthy young man, a healthy full-developed woman is thousand times more beautiful than any of them. So is a young healthy man in the eyes of a young woman. Why is it so? Because Nature wants every person to do his or her own duty of propagating his or her own species.

Both early and late marriages are injurious to health. The best time for marriage is when Nature whispers into the ears of men and women (when they have attained majority) that they are fit for reproduction by associating with a member of the opposite sex.

Suitable time for Reproduction :—When the married couple is in the best of health and spirits, and in a mood of jollity with no external circumstances to mar their pleasures, when love whispers happiness, then is the proper time for reproduction; and this should if possible coincide with the hour when all external nature is in her holiday mood and all the birds and beasts are sharing in it.

Sexual offences and Sins

Now-a-days, under the titles of "Birth Control" "Control over progeny" Limitation of families," etc., spurious books and booklets are published by doctors and even by lay people which are sold by the booksellers spuriously. With their pseudo-medical wisdom these authors make bold to recommend fraudulent means against Nature which often do great harm to those who resort to such unnatural methods. Because every deviation or departure from Nature's path is an offence against Her Laws and a sin against the moral code and it can not escape punishment from Her. The best way to control progeny is to abstain from intercourse and not to perpetrate frauds against Nature. Cold baths, fruit diet and plenty of exercise will enable one to have a control over one's passions without reducing one's strength and energy in any way.

The use of contraceptive remedies for "birth control" at will which is now-a-days recommended by many doctors and highly spoken of by many economists is a great offence against the Laws of Nature. It frustrates the object of Nature and neither party gets the natural compensation in the act; the result is premature loss of vitality and sexual wrecking. For it is merely a scientific mode of masturbation and the parties cannot escape Nature's punishment for their sexual sin as it is merely an unnatural action. Numerous persons who had practised such sexual sin consulted the author for nervousness, impotency and sexual weakness. They recovered after undergoing suitable natural mode of treatment and obeying Nature.

Intercourse during pregnancy is a serious offence against the Laws of Nature. It undermines the health of both the parties and of the unborn babe. Neither the husband nor the wife gets proper recompense and both lose their vitality slowly and surely. The child when it is born and grows up develops undue sexual irritation and in most cases turns out a masturbator.

Prostitution and adultery also are sins against the moral code and do not yield proper compensation as they are merely mercenary.

Masturbation or self abuse is a most destructive and suicidal habit dreadfully common among boys and girls, especially among those who indulge in heaty foods, narcotics, spices and stimulating drinks and among those who read love stories of low type, visit immoral cinemas or indulge in immoral and obscene talk or thoughts.

These sexual martyrs soon lose their mental and physical power and get incapacitated for marriage.

Onanism is incomplete intercourse and withdrawal of sexual organ before completing the act, for fear of such completion resulting in pregnancy. Onan was the first person known to have committed this offence, hence the word onanism is used by authors on sexual matters to indicate that offence. It is a great sin against the Laws of Nature and both the parties turn sexual, mental and physical wrecks as they do not get either proper satisfaction or compensation.

Sodomy is another most heinous offence against Nature. The perpetrators are the worst type of sexual sinners; they ultimately turn either mad or impotent.

CHAPTER V

How man the masterpiece frustrates Nature's plan and how he suffers on that account; what should he do to avoid suffering—

Man is great Nature's masterpiece
Created by her to keep peace
By governing both lands and seas
And bossing all lives which he sees.
If we survey from east to west
In this whole world he is the best
Most daring, most strong and most grand
All troubles worst he can withstand.
He can run fast, jump, ride and swim
He can shoot and kill tigers grim.
He can control beasts furious
And handle serpents venomous
Wild animals all he can tame
He can form circus from the same
And confidence in them create
To handle them with valour great.
He can climb over peaks of mounts
Worst difficulties he surmounts
No other living thing can do
All what man has done hither-to
Tide and eclipse he can predict
Things in the Mars he can depict
Can find out distance from the Sun
Can manufacture sharpest gun

Bombs he can throw, explosives spread
And can contrive machine-guns dread.
He can dig mines, can fathom seas
Build aeroplanes, climb o'er high trees
He can go e'en beyond the sea
Invisible things too he can see
He can describe the gates of hell
Its state and all its inmates fell
What's done in heaven all he can tell
As if he has surveyed it well.
Description vivid he can give
Of place where ghosts and devils live
He can talk to the persons dead
And can expound what ghosts have said
He can fight and he can argue
And prove false stories as facts true
And even facts he can disprove
Ghost's existence too he can prove
He can prove with intelligence
Almighty God's non-existence
He can make a God of a stone
By giving it a shape of his own
Or making some nice funny change
So that it may look in way strange
Or from some metal he may make
An image for his pleasure's sake
And please it with devotion great
Acts wonderful he can relate
Strange miracles he can narrate
And give out lies deliberate
Pertaining to his own strange god

And other persons thus defraud.
Though he can't show us gods in scores
He can affirm "they are in crores."
  He can prove that there are three Gods
By bringing forward pious frauds.
He can assure that God is one
And say " His favours I have won
I pleased Him with devotion strong
And prayers which I continued long."
He can impress on other's mind
That " God is merciful and kind"
But at the same time he can tell
" He has created horrid hell
To damn all those who can't believe
His Gospel but he doth relieve
Worst sinners and them doth redeem
According to his sacred scheme
If they ask pardon and repent
Such stories strange he can invent.
By blinding our good reason thus
He can try to boss all of us.
As one anointed by the High
To subjugate us he may try
He may exert both days and nights
To rob the poor their wealth and rights.
He is most shrewd, intelligent
Enduring and most deligent
He is most cunning, fraudulent
Untrustworthy and indolent
False rumours all o'er he can spread
And crocodile tears he can shed.

He can subdue enemies dread
Some hundreds of wives he can wed
His species he can propagate
At will, and can be moderate
All worst crimes he can perpetrate
And thus try to cheat Nature great.
He is most scheming, powerful
Most lustful and most beautiful
He is majestic and astute
Sublime without a substitute
He is most prudent and is wise
And can his talents exercise
All over water, air and lands
With masterly brains, eyes and hands.
But if he stupefies his brains
He suffers from worst pangs and pains
Hence poisonious drugs he should not take
His brains and health he should not stake
Great Nature's food-stuffs he must eat
And her kind bounties he must greet
He must obey her every day
Else he will suffer in worst way
With men he may frauds perpetrate
But he can't humbug Nature great.
Wise Nature is so just though kind
She favours those whom she would find
Obeying her unchanging law
Implicitly with fear and awe.
All ailments are the consequence
Of our own disobedience
To her rules and to her commands

While we fulfil our own demands
Kind Nature is supplying food
Nutritious, wholesome, fresh and good
Such as grains, nuts, herbs, milk and fruits
And vegetable green which suits
All constitutions weak and strong
In all the seasons all along
If we partake such food in-tact
We shall be free from ills in fact.
But these grains we grind well or grate
Boil them well to elaborate
And season them with troubles great
Thus fully them emasculate
Such stuff we do not masticate
Nor do we it insalivate
But swallow and leave to its fate
Our bowels first to constipate
And then severe pain to create
Or to cause colic obstinate
Producing flatus which would growl
And to cause diarrhoea foul;
Thereby some get dyspepsia
And others constant nausea
Those who thus hurriedly devour
Get eructation foul or sour
Until from such food they abstain
Or practise fast now and again.
We turn these grains in powder fine
Then heat it much to undermine
Its nutriment and make a bread
Which we bake well till it gets red

Or till it gets brown or quite black
And swallow that with wine or sack
Hence some get bad neuralgia
And others get myalgia
We do remove their husk as waste
Throw it away and change their taste
By adding spices and much salt
As if to mend great Nature's fault.
These nice grains we devide or smash
And make a hodge-podge or a mash
Or we prepare from them a cake
And on an oven hot that we bake
With mud-like liquid that we eat
Or gulp with jam or syrup sweet
Or we turn them in lumps and roast
Or we scorch them well into toast
As cooks expert though we much boast
We are no better than a ghost.

We do emasculate the rice
Removing fully its bran nice
And then by boiling completely
And voiding phosphates thoroughly
With pungent curry make a pulp
Unmasticated that we gulp
Or we boil rice with sugar sweet
Cloves, saffron and ghee and then eat
That with fried breads made up of wheat
Our tender stomach this way we treat.
There-by we get dyspepsia
Or troublesome neuralgia
Pain colic-like unbearable

Or we get thirst unquenchable
And constipation obstinate
Then intestinal looseness great.
We make hard stones and engines work
But give our own teeth chance to shirk
We don't make them food masticate
But swallow it in hurry great
We sometimes make them cold things eat
And always things producing heat
We constantly eat sugar sweet
Hence they decay or leave their seat
Thus dentists make a fortune good
Due to our errors in our food.
   Instead of chewing sugar-cane
And drinking juice as persons sane
We eat much sugar every day
Made in objectionable way.
Nuts potent we emasculate
Instead of eating in pure state
We cut them into pieces small
Add lot of salt and bake them all
Or add much sugar, make them sweet
Or fry them well before we eat.
Milk we boil to a boiling heat
To kill all microbes which take seat
In it intending to kill all
Who drink it, though they are so small
Not knowing Nature kind doth give
Us power to kill such germs and live;
If we do simply keep our blood
In pure state, it will nip in bud

All ailments by destroying such
Disease germs with a single touch;
We make milk reprehensible
And turn it indigestible
By adding sugar superfine
Its qualities we undermine
Add eggs and sugar much to change
Its taste by making custard strange;
Add spices in a way absurd
Or turn it into a sour curd
Hence strength'ning qualities all good
Milk loseth and turns worthless food
Thereby we feel intolerance
And we get oft much flatulence.
We think from ripe fruits we catch cold
And to eat them we are not bold
Green vegetable and raw fruits
And herbs we think will never suit
Our constitutions in crude state
Unless boiled well at any rate
Hence we cut them in slices thin
Add lot of spices and salt in
And boil them well in a strange way
Till their vitamines are away;
Or we add mustard, chillies, oil
And salt in them before we boil
Then swallow such stuff in hot state
And we keep blaming Nature great
As we expect nutrition good
From such emasculated food;
Hence some get scurvy obstinate

Thence pyorrhoea soon or late
Some take sweet syrup or cold drink
Or take hot drinks up to their brink
Such as tea, cocoa, coffee hot
Or chocolate hot and what not?
These substances cause nervousness
Dyspepsia and sleeplessness
Or diabetes obstinate
Then carbuncles with burning great
The stomach as a rule they dilate
Or cause its inflammation great.
Some drink much soda, gingerade
Some drink too much iced lemonade
Some drink pick-me-up, gingerale
While some take brandy, or strong ale
These substances do perforate
Internal parts cause troubles great
They always bowels constipate
And then our heart they palpitate
Some oft drink whisky, sherry fine.
And others champagne or sparkling wine,
Some smoke tobacco superfine,
Or eat it, health to undermine.
Some eat cocaine, opium
Or drugs which cause delirium
They stupefy our nerves and brains
And bring diseases in their trains.
Some oft take noxious mixture's dose
Some breathe through mouth and not through nose
These habits cause impurities
In blood and bring calamities.

Some eat fish, fowl and cattle meek
Some drink much liquor and get weak
Some don't bathe even once a week
Some fashionable wrong things seek
Thereby get pain in joints throughout
Or get sciatica or gout.
Some everload their stomach much
Till their abdomen can't bear touch
Some don't expose their skin to light
Or to fresh air to feel all right
Though Nature has meant that we should
Expose our skin in town or wood.
Some don't lie nor sit on the ground
Nor barefooted they take a round
In their own garden or in their yard
Nor on road royal smooth or hard;
The very touch of mother Earth
Would energise them and cause mirth
She may cure even all their ills
But they don't act as Nature wills.
Some promptly don't attend her call
Some oft do things unnatural
Though she is a strict sentinel
Chastising all defaulters well.
Some live in dense locality
Eat things which cause acidity
Or which cause much debility
Producing much obesity;
Take drugs which cause stupidity;
And which rob their felicity
Thus giving quacks facility

To get rich o'er calamity
Of patients for whom they don't care
To really know how they fare.
Some smell strong scents or odours strong
And get lungs spoiled by their use long
Some keep awake oft during night
And sleep in morn hence don't feel right.
Some ride on motors or on carts
Don't exercise their lower parts
Thus Nature's rules they disregard
And nourishing food they discard.
Such things not meant by her they take
And their own good health they oft stake
Then go to doctors to consult
Who drug them and cause worse result.
Drugs poisonous of any sort
Do always Nature's progress thwart;
If they check one disease at all
They do upset health natural.
One who takes drugs once in a way
Is found to take them till doom's day;
No drug, no blister nor the knife
Is needed to save human life
We can gain and preserve our health
Without expending any wealth
Obeying Nature every day
One can be healthy srong and gay.

In gloom of night and blaze of day
Grand Nature follows her own way
On creatures all she has her sway
Chastising those who go astray.

I humbly walk on her safe path
As a confirmed *Naturopath*
By solving thus her mystery
From ailments I am always free ;
I try to show to all my friends
And all the poor her ways and ends.
The healing art as exercised
By Nature great all are surprised
Obeying her plain laws with joy
The bloom of health one can enjoy
With methods simple and quite plain
The splendid health all can maintain.
Thus learned quacks with all their fame
Well versed in drugs she puts to shame.
Kind Nature wants no prayers, fee
Nor vow to be made but grants free
Her blissful bounties to the poor
As well as to the rich so sure
And safe though rich with healing powers
Which she regardless of thanks showers
Good health and cheer in every clime
Indeed are Nature's gifts sublime.
If wealth can purchase the best health
It could be owned by lords of wealth
As wealth the poor chaps can not give
They could not have been fit to live;
But we do find majority
Among the poor from ills are free
But ah ! among the lords of wealth
Minority is in good health
Thereby their doctors in the town

Roll in wealth and ride up and down
In motor or victoria
With grand paraphernalia
Good health, content and peace of mind
Are the rewards of Nature kind
For good behavior of man:
And strict obedience to plan
Immutable of Nature's own
Which she hath made to persons known
By blessing them with instinct keen
In creatures all it can be seen
Imposing e'en disorder slight
Whenever they would not act right
If they again live properly
From ailments she doth make them free.

Kulkarni hence requests you all
To please obey laws natural
Kind Nature like a mother fond
Is always ready with her wand
To pardon child undutiful
If it mends its wrong acts in full.
One can avoid all doctor's bills
By living as great Nature wills
And shunning mixtures patent pills
And drugs which are the source of ills.
Do study Nature's healing force
Its steady progress and its course
As it cures all our ailments soon
In spite of drugs it serves as boon.
Fresh air, pure water, sunlight bright

And ripe fruits can set us all right
They even do preserve one's health
Without expenditure of wealth
Employing Nature's bounties these
One can be quite free from disease.

Food cooked and uncooked

Why is disease so common and perfect health so rare? Because of errors in diet and in the mode of living. Civilization has introduced various fashions which ignore or break the laws of Nature and corrupt natural instincts of man.

Man's chief object and delight seem to be the cooking of food and mixing it with endless varieties of spices. Mixing changes the natural taste, cooking destroys the vitamines and life-sustaining and strength-giving properties, while spices make the food harmful to the general health of the consumer.

Is uncooked food less wholesome than the cooked? It is quite possible for human beings to maintain and nourish themselves on uncooked food and if properly taken it will make them healthier and stronger and keep them free from ailments.

Primitive races sustained themselves on raw and tender leaves, flowers, fruits and nuts. Famines turned them to roots and animal food, which of course required to be cooked or boiled ; later on they cultivated cereals in the rainy season and preserved them for other seasons also. These they found hard to masticate with their teeth and began to boil them well. But these cereals can be made softer by holding them in the mouth in small quantities and softening them with saliva or they may be soaked in water and made soft enough to be masticated well and swallowed after properly insalivating the liquified grains which can be digested and assimilated more easily than the cooked ones. The cereals eaten in this way will supply more nutrition, more strength and better health and even a very small quantity will suffice to sustain human life.

More than 90 percent of human ailments are caused by errors in diet *i. e.* by eating food not meant by Nature for human consumption. Uncooked food produced and ripened by Nature with the help of air, water and sunlight if properly eaten can prevent such ailments and promote health and strength and prolong life.

A few Recipes of Uncooked food.

(1) Morning—6 to 10 ounces of fresh milk
Noon—A tender cocoanut or a few plantains
Evening—6 to 8 ounces of fresh milk again

(2) Morning—A tender cocoanut
Noon—Plantains or any other fruits in season
Evening—A tender cocoanut again

(3) Morning—A handful of wheat soaked in pure water
Noon—A tender cocoanut
Evening—A handful of wheat soaked in pure water

(4) Morning—Milk and plantains
Noon—Wheat soked in water with cocoanut
Evening—Milk and plantains

(5) Morning—Wheat soaked in water with grated cocoanut
Noon—Plantains or any fruits in season
Evening—Wheat soaked in water with grated cocoanut

(6) Morning—Almonds 2 ounces soaked in water with grated cocoanut
Noon—tender cocoanut with dates
Evening—Almonds 2 ounces soaked in water with grated cocoanut

(7) Morning—Milk with dates
Noon—tender cocoanut
Evining—milk with dates

---

(1) Morning—Sesame with milk
Noon—Dates with tender cocoanut
Evening—Sesame with milk

(2) Morning—Dates with grated cocoanut
Noon—Sesame with plantains
Evening—Dates with grated cocoanut

(3) Morning—pistachio with milk
Noon—Tender cocoanut
Evening—pistachio with milk

(4) Morning—Almonds with dates
Noon—Tender cocoanut
Evening—Almond and dates

(5) Morning—Milk with dates
Noon—Sesame with cocoanut
Evening—Milk with dates

(6) Morning—Walnuts, dates and grated cocoanut
Noon—plantains and any fruits in season
Evening—Walnuts, dates and grated cocoanut

(7) Morning—Milk with almonds
Noon—Tender cocoanut
Evening—Milk and almonds

---

(1) Morning—Milk and honey
Noon—Dates and cocoanuts
Evening—Milk and honey

(2) Morning—Milk and dates
Noon—Cocoanuts and honey
Evening—Milk and figs

(3) Morning—Milk and figs
Noon—Cocanuts and dates
Evening—Milk and almonds

(4) Morning—sesame and dates
Noon—Cocoanut and figs
Evening—sesame and dates

(5) Morning—Milk, bananas, kajunuts.
Noon—Cocoanut and dates
Evening—Milk bananas and nuts

(6) Morning—Cocoanut with sesame
Noon—Plantains and dates
Evening—Milk, and sesame

(7) Morning—Milk and plantains
Noon—Cocoanuts and dates
Evening—Milk and plantains

All cereals must be eaten fresh before they dry up. In the absence of fresh ones dried ones must be soaked in pure water.

(1) Morning—Milk and any cereals
Noon—Tender cocoanuts with dates or figs
Evening—Milk and cereals

(2) Morning—Milk and figs
Noon—Cocoanuts and dates
Evening—Milk and figs or cereals

(3) Morning—Milk and dates dried
Noon—Tender cocoanuts and grapes
Evening—Milk and dates or cereals

(4) Morning—Milk and plantains
Noon—Cocoanut and grapes
Evening—Milk and plantains

(5) Morning—Milk, *sesame* and dates
Noon—Cocoanut, grapes or dates
Evening—Milk, *sesame* and dates

(6) Morning—Milk and apples or plantains
Noon—Cocoanut, dates or figs
Evening—Milk, apples or plantains

(7) Morning—Milk with cereals
Noon—Cocoanut with dates or grapes
Evening—Milk with cereals

Recipes of uncooked food for those who like varieties and mixtures of several foodstuffs

(1) Morning—Plate No. 1—plantain, cut into slices, grated tender cocoanut with little honey.
Noon—Any cereals with almonds or cocoanut
Evening—Same as morning

(2) Morning—Plate No. 2— Milk and honey with almonds or cocoanut

Noon—Tomatoe slices with grated cocoanut and sliced onion with lemon juice and coriander leaves

Evening—Same as morning

(3) Morning—Milk with almond, pistachio and *charoli*

Noon—Plate No. 3—grated tender cocoanut with cucumber slices and onion slices with honey or lemon juice or both

Evening—Same as morning

(4) Morning—Milk and honey with a little powdered nutmeg or cardamom

Noon—Plate No. 4—tender cocoanut, tender lady's fingers cut into slices, onion slices with honey or lemon juice or both

(5) Morning—Milk and honey with very little saffron

Noon—Plate No. 5—cocoanut, beetroot slices with honey or lemon juice or both

Evening—Same as morning

(6) Morning—Milk and honey with cardamom

Noon—Plate No. 6—cocoanut slices, carrots, sliced onion with honey or lemon juice

Evening—Same as morning

(7) Morning—Milk with honey and pistachio

Noon—Plate No. 7—grated cocoanut, slices of radish and onion with lemon juice

Evening—Same as morning

Different kinds of dishes may be prepared from tender sprouts of any green vegetable, flower petals, cucumbers of different varieties, and all green and fresh vegetables in season. Rose petals will relieve constipation while pomegranate petals will cure loose motions.

Food stuffs of different sorts may be prepared from cereals before they are well dried.

If undried ones are not available, dried ones may be soaked in water for some hours and used as food with grated cocoanut, onion slices and lemon juice.

Berries of different varieties may be eaten alone or with tender cocoanut, dates, figs or any other dried and preserved fruits.

Fruits such as mangoes, jack fruits, peaches, fresh figs, kaju fruits, etc. may be freely used and are very wholesome if they are eaten in their season.

Nuts of different kinds fresh or preserved by drying when masticated well, insalivalted properly, and eaten, supply nutrition and strength and preserve natural health. If teeth are not strong enough the nuts may be soaked in pure water and eaten.

Syrups and cold drinks for hot season.

Tender cocoanut juice is the best drink both to quench the thirst and also to serve as a general tonic as it contains so many nutritive bio-chemic phosphates and chlorides which are needed for the human blood.

Sugar-cane pieces when chewed well yield juice which satiate thirst in hot season and also during fevers. The juice serves also as a general tonic and an effective cure for flatulence and dyspepsia.

Juices squeezed fresh from sour lemons, sweet limes, oranges, pomegranets, apples, mangoes, jack fruits, kaju fruits, etc. and mixed in required quantity with pure water and sipped in small quantities serve as excellent fresh syrups. If desired a little honey to sweeten and a little powder of nutmeg or cardamom may be added for flavouring.

Whenever there is constipation, yellow lemon juice and sweetlime juice are preferable, and when the stools are loose pomegranet juice is preferable.

For scanty urine radishes, sweet limes, lemons, *punarnava* leaves, coriander leaves, dil leaves or fennel leaves may be squeezed in pure water and taken with honey or sour lemon juice or with both.

Vegetable substitutes for flesh-meat preparations.

A decoction prepared from the slices of *Bhendies* known as Ladys fingers is an excellent substitute for beef-tea, mutton soup, chicken-soup, Virol, Bovril and other preparations of animal flesh, bones, etc. Uncooked cocoanut and slices of *Bhendies* and onion mixed are an excellent plate both as food and tonic. A little honey or lemon juice may be added for taste.

Cocoanut milk *i. e.* its juice is far superior to cod liver oil and so many of its preparations sold by chemists.

Cocoanut juice rubbed over the limbs and spine is a better substitute for pancreatic emulsion or cod liver-oil in case of rickets.

Decoction prepared from carrots and beet roots with a little honey is an excellent substitute for Hemotogen, Hemoglobin, etc. prescribed by doctors for anaemia.

Chest-nuts, violet coloured brinjals, china-bread, (fruit known as *Divi panas,*) sweet potatoes, potatoes with onions are excellent substitutes for so many flesh meat preparations. They taste better and supply better nutrition than meat preparations.

If all people will have recourse to the above diet, all ailments and diseases will disappear like shadows before the sun and doctors and chemists will alike find their occupation gone. There will be perfect health and harmony and there will be no offences against Nature such as masturbation, adultery, prostitution, dissipation, alcoholism, etc. nor any desire to commit theft, suicide or homicide and this whole world will be like a bed of roses without a thorn.

CHAPTER VI.

Statement of a learned man and the advice thereof by the author

I feel pain in my lower part
Which makes me travel by a cart
The nature of pain is so smart
From joint to joint it doth depart
It does not give me rest nor sleep
But it oft makes me moan and weep.
I live in this Ward's Eastern parts
I am a Bachelor of Arts.
In this grand University
I've studied Electricity
Both ancient modern History
And In-organic Chemistry
I have learnt Trigonometry
With Algebra, Geometry
Both Euclid's and new Practical,
And Languages dead Classical
Both Botany, Zoonomy
Heat and Light and Astronomy
These I have studied properly
And finished with skill masterly
An up-to-date Geography
And Logic and Philosophy
Both Grammar and Philology
With Physics and Biology
I studied with an ardent zeal
And thus spread my fame a good deal;
All what I could I have explored

And choicest books all I have stored
All poems fine I know by heart
I am well known for painter's Art
Both wisdom and skill having shown
I have become all over known.

But my head aches, my sight gets dim
My mind feels weary full of whim
I always put on this thick pair
Of spectacles, as I can't bear
This dazzling sun light and its glare
Hence my eyes I do not lay bare.
In vertex as if it would tear
I feel sharp pain which I cant bear
I get pain shooting in right ear
While my both ears refuse to hear
I feel pain supra-orbital
Which robs me of my comforts all
My gums emit pus or they bleed
And I cant eat the food I need
All my fine teeth do always shake
And some of them at times so ache
My tongue is blistered and turned red
And can't bear touch of finest bread
I feel great craving for strong tea
And coffee hot which I drink free
I do drink Soda, Lemonade
Or Pick-me-up or Gingerade
Rum, Brandy, Whiskey, liquor fine
Champagne, Gin, Sherry or strong wine
Such beverages I do drink

At times too much up to my brink
To drink cold water I'm not bold
As I at once catch nasty cold
To overcome that tendency
I smoke tobacco frequently
I use cigars and *Birds-eye* fine
Though health they seem to undermine.
I can't digest milk, *Ghee* and wheat
Breads, biscuits and cakes I cant eat
Jams, chutneys, pickles I do take
Though they are causing frequent ache
In my weak stomach which doth crave
Strong liquors and they make me brave
Intoxication makes me rave
When sober I feel half in grave.
My weak heart doth oft palpitate
My bowels always constipate
In liver I feel awful pain
To pass hard stools I always strain
At times I do pass foul profuse
With griping, dreadful motions loose
In my abdomen flatus foul
Whenever I eat or drink doth growl
In fearful way as it would burst
My belly or cause colic worst.
In Kidneys I feel pain at night
In urine I pass small threads white
At times I pass albumin much
Or sediments or some stuff such
My urine is oft passed in drops
And burns the parts or at times stops

At times I pass it copious
And feel for that state piteous
My toes and fingers and my neck
Get shooting pain which I can't check
Though special care I always take
My muscles and large joints all ache
Skin gets itch and eruptions dread
Which I scratch much till it gets red
I do not get sleep during night
Nor during day to feel all right
Though I feel drowsy I do keep
Awake without a wink of sleep
I frequently get fever high
Which sometimes makes me moan and sigh
I can't bear hot sun nor wind rough
Exposure least doth cause me cough
But I cant bring up any stuff
Though I make efforts long enough;
I suffer so much in this way
Though I wear flannel the whole day.
A doctor great I did consult
Expecting soon a good result
Who gave me drugs to make me purge
Not to do so though I did urge
They drove my state from bad to worse
For which my own luck I do curse;
He then gave me expectorants
Some tonics and some stimulants
Quinine and Morphine he then gave
They made my state more and more grave

Consulting then experts of west
He got examined my tongue, chest
Heart, urine and blood and did his best
But they could not give me good rest.
These specialists of high repute
Could not improve my ills acute
As ailments all then took worse form
Instead of showing some reform.
As last resource health to repair
They recommended change of air;
Though a place healthy I did choose
It did not prove of any use.
Then I went to a famous *Vaid*[1]
" I can cure in one week " he said
And talked of *humours* like a quack
Felt my pulse, liver, heart and back
And said " your nerves are very slack "
And opened then his mystic sack
Took out some pills and made me eat
And said "lot of sick men I treat
If you eat these pills for a week
You will be strong and won't feel weak
Your health these pills will soon restore
And you won't feel pains any more
These are made up of mercury
Gold, sulphur and rich *Kastury*[2]
These are unfailing tonic pills
They can cure all sorts of worst ills
They do all *Doshas*[3] pacify

---

1. Ayurvedic physician; 2. Musk 3. Humours.

And human bodies fortify"
But they caused a good deal of heat
And I could not sit on my seat
They did inflame my body whole
And did torment the inner soul
I thought then he was paving way
To heaven thus to send me away
This world then as I could not leave
My pains as he could not relieve
I wished him thus a last Good-bye
And elsewhere went my luck to try.
Next I went to an *Unany*
Hakeem to try my destiny
Well-known experienced and wise
Who doth dispense drugs in sweet guise
In shape of syrups valued high
Which even kings and *Nababs* try
All noble *Begums*[1], *Ranees*[2] too
Do prefer them to nectar true.
"My medicated special *Jams*"
He said "were tried by *Sabs*[3] and *Ma'ams*
And highly praised and much approved
Their efficacy is thus proved
By grace of *Allah* I am sure
The life despaired e'en to ensure
And raise the dying from death bed
Though doctors them declare as dead;
These doctors and these surgeons great
Can excellently operate
They are more skilful and more bold

1. Mohamedan queens 2. Hindu queens 3. Sahibs.

Than non-diplomaed surgeons old
But in such sweet drugs they don't deal
Worst ailments with these I can heal;
The opulent in Northern Hind
From Bengal East to Western Sind
Have tried and they know them full well
As these relieved their ills like spell."
But in my case they did not prove
Of use as they could not improve
My shattered health in any way
But made me suffer night and day.
  Then I had to come back again
To doctors for relief of pain
One after one I did try then
Some specialists and famous men
One thought it was good to remove
My blood through leeches and improve
My pains neuralgic and did bleed
But that made me more weak indeed
Though that gave me a short relief
On the whole it increased my grief
His action thus shook my belief
In bleeding process even brief.
The other ordered liquid food
He said "No other will do good"
He recommended broth and soup
Both my health and strength to recoup
They couldn't in any way decrease
My pains, but rather did increase.
I was in a dilemma great
When one prescribed me in this state

To try enema moderate
My intestines to regulate
I didn't comply with his command
As he had no diploma grand
And in this state of health I had
Great fear of getting dropsy bad.
Another one tried "*six naught six*"
That did put me in a great fix
An awful ordeal it was
A dreadful burning it did cause
From my head up, down to my toe
And thus it did increase my woe.
Another doctor thought it best
That I should take a perfect rest
And should not move from my sick bed
Till I felt well or I was dead.
Though it seemed to me trivial
It was a funny ordeal
As it made stiff my every joint
And made me worse in every point.
The next tried Electricity
Which made worse my calamity
By making all my joints quite loose
And weak like those of an old goose
Though it gave me relief at first
It later on made my pains worst.
One said " By using Guilotine
an remove your tonsils fine
easy method I now choose
y seem to be of no use
ds and coughs thus I can cure

Without drugs in ten days be sure"
Another says "I shall remove
Appendix, your health to improve
As lavish Nature is a fool
I am informed so in my school
Removing thus the seat of pain
Relief for you I can obtain"
The last one says "you won't improve
Unless a dentist will remove
All your teeth and fix a set new"
Which is the latest course he knew
He says "this measure does not fail"
But I know it's of no avail
A friend whose teeth are thus removed
Is not in any way improved;
Without a tooth and a moustache
With pains rheumatic, water-brash
And with nephritis and brain fag
My friend now looks like an old hag.
These dentists and these doctors too
Have no appreciation true
Of natural teeth and our health
They all try to increase their wealth
I want to know opinion fair
What shall I do in this affair
I have become a perfect wreck
Of former self now with stiff neck,
Lumbago, cramps, neuralgia,
Foul flatus and dyspepsia;
With Morphia and Aspirin
My ailments now he tries to win ;

They make my muscles weak and soft
And do cause palpitation oft
Professing my own self as wise
I have gone in "*Fool's Paradise*"
Though I was the pride of my shool
I think "*I am a greatest fool*"
As I have lost all peace of mind
With all my thoughts and acts refined
Whether I go out, sit in room
Or chat with friends I feel all gloom
All what I learnt and what I knew
Now seems to me bosh and untrue
This is my sad and awful tale
Which doth make me oft weep and wail.
In colleges what is now taught
and what we learn there, is not fraught
With knowledge useful for our health
It tends to lose one's health and wealth.
In all the classes primary
Health rules should he compulsory
And on all obligatory
Authorities should teach them free
Laws hygienic they must teach
And gospel of health they must preach
They culture physical should choose
Instead of subjects of no use.
The present students are much weak
Their heavy studies make them meek
Before they finish their hard course
They lose all energy and force
Thus they can not have some resource

For their bread to find out some source
Some suffer from long sleeplessness
While others get much nervousness
Most of them get much haughtiness
And others lose their happiness
And almost all get their sight weak
While all some stimulant drugs seek
As a result they get disease
Then in worse poisons they seek ease.
The rich consult then some M. D.
While the poor take no remedy
They rather suffer quietly
As doctors charge them heavily
In charitable hospital
They are not treated well at all
In public small dispensaries
They get increased their miseries
As they are first purged frequently
And then given strong drugs carelessly
At least they say such is their state
Hence they do not try there their fate
Both doctor's fees and chemist's charge
For noxious drastic doses large
The poor can not afford to pay
From mixtures hence they keep away.
They try Homoeopathic pills
Or some decoctions for their ills
Still I find the poor student's state
Far better than that of rich mate
Great many a such candidate
Is oft seen with dress up-to-date

With spectacles they may be seen
All over the town's pensive scene
Contaminating atmosphere
With smoke of cigars everywhere
There with a match box they make trips
And hold fine cigars in their lips
Some are seen with petitions long
And bottles of drugs smelling strong
Most of them are seen in the street
As officers them do not greet
They do not like these candidates
Though fashionable graduates
In work, old staff they can't excel
Though they are educated well
They do demand high salary
Though they possess no energy
While studying they have spent much
So they expect to earn sums such
With western pomp and luxuries
They are all full of miseries
As they can't earn big salaries
To gratify necessities;
They are in such a wretched state
Though they long for position great.
I think I am worst in the lot
With all my comforts I have got
Though I am rich I have no rest
And peace, though I longed for all best.
All my ambitions I have lost
And now wish to pay any cost
If I could get a peaceful end

He who grants it is my best friend
A poor man leading wretched life
I think is happy with his wife
The children of the working class
Without an ailment their days pass
Why God Almighty kind and just
Should in this way be so unjust
Why should I suffer such worst pain
Though I take drugs now and again
Consulting doctors of repute
Skilled in ills chronic and acute.
Though I am only thirtyfive
For five years more I may not thrive
'Tis better to pass my last breath
Than to live such a living death
Of what an earthly good is wealth
To me who can't possess good health
As last resource I wish to try
Your healing method or to die
As it is spoken of so high
By a friend of mine by-the-bye.

Advice thereof by the author

Contentment, peace and perfect health
Are far superior to wealth
Ranks, degrees, titles and grand dress
One's grievances do not redress
To mind unripe they cause false pride
And make it Nature's ways deride
Thus easily it falls a prey

Soon to deceiptful Fashion's sway
Like a kid silly in new guise
To vixen vigilant and wise
Obeying Nature day by day
You must find out redemption's way
Her method does not fascinate
Like Fashion's tempting charming bait
Her ways and methods do not tempt
But everyday you must attempt
And follow her way like a meek
And humble child to comforts seek
Though she is just she is so kind
Like a fond mortal mother's mind
Her mind is ready to forgive
Her child, if it begins to live
A simple life as she intends
And all its crooked ways it mends.
Vile Fashion is like Satan fell
She doth tempt and sends one to hell
The best way is her to discard
And always be on one's own guard
Kind Nature is a mother just
While Fashion a wench full of lust
With youthful gestures decked with gold
More pleasing than the mother old
Who is just with commanding tone
But she can all your sins atone.
Do follow her steps as a mild
Obedient and humble child
Her free gifts with work and repose
Can save you from the doctor's dose

Fresh air, pure water, sun light bright,
Ripe fruits and exercise though light
Will gradually set you right
By putting all your ills to flight.
That one deserves my high respect
Who says " All fashions I neglect
Great Nature's ways I don't oppose
Or as a grand man I don't pose
Through Nature ailments I have wun
All food not meant by her I shun "
There is no need of mixtures, pills,
And doctors grand e'en in worst ills
Their mixtures of drugs poisonous
Have played more havoc all round us
Than ailments themselves of all kind
The fact is known to thoughtful mind.
Do not take Morphine, Opium
Nor Bromide of potassium
To bring you on refreshing sleep
Away from such drugs you must keep
A hot foot-path or warm full bath
And your foot-steps on Nature's path
Will soon enable you at night
To sleep well and to feel all right.
At night if you do not get sleep
Then brooding over do not keep
A hot foot bath short if you take
You will sleep till morn and won't wake.
If bowels yours do constipate
To take purgatives you must hate
As they do always cause worse state

In cases such you should not wait
But should take an enema soon
It serves well in time as a boon
A shower bath on head and spine
And neck is a good plan of mine
It doth prevent neuralgic pain
And from it one can vigonr gain.
Tic, migrane, prosopalgia
Neuralgia, myalgia
All will be driven far away
By shower bath in a fine way.
Don't take Phenalgin, Aspirin
Phenacetin nor saccharin
Don't take cocaine, coca wine
Nor any liquors superfine
They have caused more mortality
Than ills with taciturnity
Than wars and famines of worst type
And cholera with purge and gripe
Than erysipelas of head
And pestilence with buboes dread
Believe not quack's nor doctor's fuss
And never take drugs poisonous
Do not be tempted by the praise
Of chemists who intend to raise
The value of some doctor's make
Their efforts are for Mammon's sake
If doctors praise some chemists grand
Who deal in drugs of poison brand
Be sure those drugs you do not need
They do all that for their own greed.

Fresh air, pure water, work and rest
And sunlight are the healers best
Baths simple and food natural
Can cure pains and diseases all.
Away from Nature's path you are
As you have deviated far
You must return to Nature kind
And then you will have peace of mind
You have been trying to defraud
Kind Nature and Almighty God
By leading life unnatural
Hence you should not blame them at all.
If you obey Her with your heart
And soul, all your ills will depart
As all ills are the consequence
Of your own wholesale negligence
Of her resources which you had
Made all these years to cause health bad.
Obeying Nature kind again
You can cure worst disease and pain.
From liquors, coffee and strong tea.
And wines you must be always free
Rum, brandy, whisky you don't drink
To drink wines also you must shrink
Be satisfied with Adam's ale
As it will surely make you hale
You can eat ripe fruits in good lot
But should not take food or drink hot
Do not take syrup nor drinks cold
From acid drinks you must withhold
Ripe fruits are best for quenching thirst

When thirsty you must eat them first.
Do not eat pickles, salted food
Nor spices as they don't do good
You should avoid fish, fowl and meat
And be content with milk and wheat
Green vegetables you may eat
But don't eat sweetmeats and jams sweet.
Do not eat custard and things fried
Nor any thing preserved or dried
Do not take any drink or food
Which in fact can not do you good
When you feel hungry you may take
Food nutritive for your health's sake
Your stomach is not a *go down*
Where foods, drinks and drugs can be thrown
In any way or as you like
Until it feels tired and would strike
To do its duty being weak
And other measures it would seek
Such as cramps, colic, heart-burn, pain
Or constipation causing strain
Or diarrhoea to relieve
Its burden for which you would grieve
Or it might vomit the food or bile
And thus decline to reconcile
Till you give it a perfect rest
And it feels able to digest
All natural supply of food
To human beings which does good;
All poisons and drugs you must shun
Keep merry with songs, wit and fun

Walk always on great Nature's path
Twice every day take a sun bath
And hip bath only once a day
You will improve in a fine way.
You should mend all your actions wrong
Should not keep smoking all along
In daily habits do not cope
With learned persons of Europe
All Eastern methods don't discard
Though they seem to you strange and hard
Discretion always you must use
And good things from both you must choose
There lies your wisdom and your tact
And that will give you peace in fact.
Try to avoid sleep during day
T to be always bright and gay
An be contented in your mind
To every living thing be kind
Take morning walks in sunlight bright
Wear white clothes and take rest at night
Keep always working during noon
Thereby you will improve health soon
A merry heart and peaceful mind
Save us from worries of all kind
You need not get your teeth removed
But daily see your bowels are moved
Digestve organs if work well
Excretions all if you expel
And if blood is kept always pure
Diseases all you can soon cure.
To lead a simple life you try

Don't use oil scented nor hair dye
Do not get smothered with neck-tie
And elevated collar high
Do not wear hats with leather line
Nor a big turban coloured fine
Let nature's gifts *fresh air* and *light*
Touch head and neck and make them bright
Man should expose to light and air
His head and skin by laying bare
Great Nature's this established rule
We should not try to over-rule
To men in towns though it looks strange
Great Nature's law we can not change
Unless we pay it's penalty
Of losing our vitality ;
Don't keep a pigtail nor shave head
You can have a fine crop instead
Do not shave your lips to look fine
Disfiguring face masculine
Don't wear tight clothes and suffocate
All pores which will cause troubles great
To your lungs and your kidneys too
As they are their partakers true
Do not wear flannel and coats tight
Wear porous clothes of cotton white
Let sunlight your clothes penetrate
And fresh air your pores ventilate
They surely will make your blood pure
And all diseases they will cure
They may help even kidneys too
As skin performs their functions true

Do not squeeze your feet in boots tight
Expose them well to air and light
Wash them well whene'er they get soiled
But do not have their structure spoiled
In morn do stretch both of your hands
Inhale fresh air till chest expands
And then exhale quite steadily
Do sixteen times thus properly
Repeat this in noon and at eve
All troubles it can soon relieve
This will all your blood oxidise
And your whole system energise.
We can live well without a chair
Or cot so long we get fresh air
Without a table, pots and cooks
Without coats, pants, shirts, hats and books
Without ghee, spices, eggs and meat
Without salt, sugar, rice and wheat
Without a frying pan to fry
Without a soap and barber sly
One can be happy hale and strong
And having no cares can live long;
One can live e'en without a house
But not without fruits, water, spouse
As these are one's needs natural
Supplied by Nature to suit all
With these own life one can maintain
And multiply now and again
One's species own in a fine way
And in accord with Nature's sway;
She doth implant a strong desire

In living beings to respire
And appetites to gratify
And all their wants to satisfy
But we behave against her will
Our own desires we don't fulfil
In natural way and get ill
And thus keep paying doctor's bill
We disobey her frequently
And cannot therefore happy be
Man is no doubt a prodigy
Of Nature with great energy
Skill, power, strength and intelligence
If he lives well with deligence
By using properly his sense
He can rise to great prominence;
He can command all beasts of prey
As a lord he can all survey
He can be free from all disease
And he can pass his days with ease
But he much hankers after wealth
And disregards all laws of health
He swallows always too much food
Which in no way can do him good
He goes on gulping patent pills
And doctor's mixtures, pays his bills
Who keeps him in gross ignorance
Of Nature's laws and dulls his sense
By giving him drugs more and more
Which as a rule do not restore
His shattered health but make it worse
While they help to fill doctor's purse.

And to enrich his chemist sly
With cunning methods who doth try
To force down poisons in your throat
By putting over them a sweet coat;
He tries his best not to disclose
His poisonous and harmful dose
Defrauding thus our tongue and nose
Lives human slowly he doth close
Both doctors, chemists thus combine
Our splendid health to undermine.
We should not allow a single mote
To pass in stomach through our throat
Unless by eyes and nose approved
And by both tongue and teeth improved
What we eat we should masticate
And properly insalivate
Then only it should pass through throat
And not with a sweet sugar coat
What is unsightly do not eat
Foul smelling stuff you should not greet
Distasteful foods you should not crave
As they will hurry you to grave
Don't think these sugar coated pills
Are suitable to cure your ills
Defrauding thus your eyes and nose
And tongue don't gulp unpleasant dose
Your stomach such dose can't tolerate
It will soon cause you troubles great
Such as thrush, stomatitis, sprue
Or scurvy, pyorrhoea too
Foul flatus, ulcer, cancer bad

Which will soon or late make you sad
Drugs poisonous you should not take
As they will always your health stake
Kind Nature's fresh supply of food
Will only always do you good
She surely can make you quite free
From ailments all and misery
Hence study Her laws and progress
For troubles all she can redress.
Teeth, tonsils and appendix too
Their proper functions have to do
Depriving organs these be sure
That one can't proper cure ensure
By thus removing organs these
Don't think they can your ills appease
One ailment thus if they control
They cause some other on the whole
Be sure that e'en a hair on skin
Is safeguarding the part within
It hydrogen doth separate
And carbon it doth liberate
By shaving and removing hair
We may think that we look more fair;
But the removal of hair thus
Doth cause harm and disfigures us
Obeying Nature kind again
You can be free from ills and pain
Mind no fad theological
Nor social whims nor medical
Be clean in body pure in mind
And true in actions of all kind.

Kind Nature you are not to pray
Nor any sum to her you pay
But her laws you have to obey
Implicitly both night and day
Behaving thus in simple way
You can be happy, hale and gay
Good health and cheer in every clime
Indeed are Nature's gifts sublime
By making free use of air, light
And water you can be all rigt.
  The learned patient who heard all
My hints led a life natural
Observing all instructions these
He soon obtained a perfect ease
Vis Medicatrix Naturae
From ailments all she makes us free
Obeying Nature every day
We can be healthy, strong and gay.

CHAPTER VII.

इदं गुह्यतमं ज्ञानं प्रवक्ष्यामि हिताय ते।
यज्ज्ञात्वा मोक्ष्यसे रोगादारोग्यं लभसे ध्रुवम् ॥

I give this profoundest of secrets for thy welfare, by knowing which thou wilt be free from disease and attain perpetual health.

The Five Great Constituents

Of our body of which the Universe is composed of; What they achieve in our body

In the Vedant Philosophy of the Hindus it is said that the universe in its present state is the result of evolution. Vedantists do not believe that it was created out of "*nothing*". They say that out of स्वयंभू *Swayambhu* the self existing आत्मा *Atma* universal soul आकाश *Akasha* the aether evolved. This aether is invisible to the human eye like वायु *wayu* the wind. It occupies the whole universe and in which all the stars and planets float. From that aether originated वायु the wind which with its frictions produced अग्नि *Agni*, the fire. Heat of the fire combined with the wind gave birth to water, out of which sprang the solid mass of the suns, stars, comets and planets including our earth. This earth surrounded by the atmosphere and moistened by water gave birth to trees and creepers spontaneously when heated by the sun. These plants bore foodstuffs such as fruits, nuts and germinating seeds from which the whole animal kingdom took its birth with its power of propagating its own species. And प्रकृति or

Nature is the cause of all this; and this all pervading Nature still governs every thing in this universe.

एतस्मादात्मनः—आकाशः सम्भूतः
आकाशाद्वायुः—वायोरग्निः
अग्नेरापः—अद्भ्यः पृथिवी
पृथिव्याः-औषधयः । औषधीभ्यः—अन्नम्
अन्नाद्रेतः—ततः प्रजाः

Thus the matter of which this universe is composed is in five forms; they are known as *Panchabhootas* or five primary elements or substances.

(1) आकाश *Akasha*, the aether though सर्वव्यापी, all-pervading, is invisible and is to be known by our intellect only.

(2) वायु *Wayu*, the wind is *Chalanapara i. e.* characterised by motion (Sanskrit वा wä to move) and is known by our sense of touch.

(3) अग्नि *Agni* the fire is characterised by its heat and illuminating power and is known by our sight and touch.

(4) आप: *Apa* the water is liquid (which can be turned into gaseous and solid forms also) and is known from our sight and touch.

(5) पृथिवी the earth is dense, hard and firm and is known by our sight and touch.

These are the primary differentiations of cosmic matter in the universe.

Our bodies are formed of these 5 elements:—they are known as भू, जल, तेज, समीर, ख.

(1) भू or earth substance in our body is highly refined and organised into 12 tissue salts which are found in the ashes of the human body even after cremation. (For full particulars see the author's Biochemic Guide and Biochemic Prescriber.)

Mud and clay compresses have been now used frequently by some Naturopaths. Even Adolph Just cites some clinical cases. But the author had no occasions to try any himself, though he observed the results where others have tried them. They have produced no better results than Hydropathic compresses. Further they always impede the functions of the pores wherever they are used, and the author does not approve of them as they are not in accord with Nature's process of healing. They often irritate the skin when the ingredients are not pure. The earthly matter in the human body is highly refined into inorganic cellsalts and Dr. Schuessler's Boichemistry clearly shows which of those cell-salts is needed in what ailment. Pure water medicated with those suitable salts produces marvellous results, when used as compress even in all sorts of worst diseases. Therefore the author recommends the use of those cellsalts freely for use as compress instead of those dirty mud and clay compresses. (See Biochemic Prescriber by the author).

The author has however tried a sand-compress over a small area and also fomentation of sand heated in the hot sun or a hot oven when sunlight was not available over abdomen in flatulent colic and on some painful boils with good results.

(2) जल or watery substance plays an imporıant part in our body both in upkeeping and restoring health; for full details—(see "*Scientific Hydropathy*" a detailed treatise on watercure on scientific principles by the author).

तेज—The sun's substance which we have in us is the very heat, life and soul of living beings. It also plays a very important part in both preserving and regaining our health. (For full details see author's "Practical Chromopathy or Helio-therapy")

Sunlight.

The influence of sunligh upon the vital processes has been recognized from the earliest times. The old Greeks and Romans employed the sun-bath or insolation very frequently in the treatment of chronic maladies of all sorts. The natives of the South sea Islands and other primitive peoples still utilise this powerful agent in the treatment of the sick. The natives of the *Terre celiente* of Mexico have long practised exposure to Sunlight on the sea-beach partially covered with sand, as a treatment for syphilis, the patients thus treated being made to drink large quantities of infusions of leaves of various sorts while exposed to the sun The natives of Haiti are said by M. Delow to employ similar practices. (Kellogg).

All physicians place the highest value upon exposure to the sun by an out of door life as a means of stimulating the nutritive processes of the body in many chronic disorders such as anaemia, tuberculosis, and in convalescence from fevers and other similar condition.

The value of the *Sunbath* as a therapeutic measure will be readily appreciated by noting the facts respecting its remarkable physiological influence which must be very largely attributed to the actinic rays although a share of it must be attributed to the calorific effect of the Sun's rays (Kellogg). The sunbath is a more valuable and practical exciting measure; it owes its properties to the three sets of rays of which it is composed *viz.* thermal, luminous and actinic or chemical rays. The thermal and luminous rays are direclly stimulating to the cells of the tissues, causing a development and accumulations of heat while the actinic rays act upon the nervous system in a most powerful manner.

The Sun-bath or Insolation.

Sunlight is one of the most powerful of all hygienic and curative agents. As a hygienic measure it is of inesteemable value in the destruction of dangerous microbes, most of which are unable to resist the action of the direct rays of the Sun for more than a few minutes. Sunlight is thus the most important of all disinfecting and sterilising agencies. The value of sunlight in the maintenance of health is well shown in the dwarfed development or rapid deterioration of plants deprived of its stimulating influence. In caves, mines and other places from which the light is excluded plants with the exception of the fungi do not grow or if they do, very quickly die never attaining maturity. Animals also are dwarfed and become sickly under these conditions (Kellogg). In hospitals a larger percentage of recoveries occurs on the sunny side than on the shady side of the ward.

Physiological effects—The sun's rays not only influence the skin, but pass through the skin into the body exciting and stimulating the cells and tissues. The surface circulation is greatly accelerated, free perspiration occurs, the heart's action is increased and the activity of all the vital functions is promoted. In many cases the patient experiences very pronounced sensations of langour and drowsiness during the bath and not infrequently falls asleep. The effects of the Sun-bath are practically identical with those of the electric light-bath. Sunlight may be properly regarded as not only a source of radiant energy in the form of heat but as a powerful tonic through its actinic rays. Its calorific or heating rays may be isolated by placing a red glass screen between the Sun and the patient so that the actinic rays are filtered out. For tonic effects, the caloric rays may be separated by employing a blue glass screen in like manner.

Sun bath is taken by lying on a mat in a perfectly nude state and by exposing the whole body to sunlight. Sensitive persons who get headache or who feel dizziness may protect their heads with a large green leaf, preferably of a plantain tree or any other plant or with a wet cloth of green or blue colour. It should be taken for a period from 30 to 60 minutes or even longer till the patient perspires freely. After sun-bath he should take a hip bath to cool the system and it should be followed by a brisk walk in the sun to have reaction and to obtain normal temperature of the body. The best time for a sunbath is from 10 A. M. to 3 P. M. Those who are not accustomed to it should, in the beginning, take sun-bath in the mild sunlight only.

Partial sun baths—These are taken with the best results in case of nodules, tumours, indurations, painful parts, interal or external growths, ulcers, open sores, boils, abscesses, carbuncles, cancers, etc. The author has tried sun baths directly or through green or blue glasses in such diseases and found even the worst pain of cancer eased by it. He has also given sun bath to the abdomen of typhoid patients with best results. Diarrhoea, dysentary, tabes mesenterica have yielded very satisfactorily to these sun baths when judiciously administered to the abdomen of such patients.

Therapetuic applications—The sunbath is useful in all cases of malnutrition, anæmia, inactivity of the skin, chronic dyspepsia, worst cases of neurasthenia, indigestion, chlorosis, rheumatism, diabetes and obesity. (Kellogg). The ancient made great use of the sunbath in the treatment of the sick. According to Plutarch, Diogenes, the renowned Athenian cynic, was in his old age accustomed to lie in the sunshine for the purpose of recruiting his energies, a custom which according to Pliny was common among the old men in Greece. It is stated that Diogenes valued his sunbath so highly that when called upon by Alexander who offered to render him any service in his power he replied, "Only stand a little out of my sunshine". (Kellogg).

Caution—Those who are not accustomed to sunbath are likely to get sunstroke or heat stroke if they are exposed to strong light for a long time. Such sensitive persons should expose themselves only for five minutes in the beginning and the duration should be increased gradually to one to two hours. The head must be protected with green leaves and the body must be protected with a green or blue sheet made wet if necessary.

(4) वायु the wind—The Importance of wind as a constituent *i. e.* essential substance in our body for the preservation of life has already been mentioned in detail in this book. See chapters I, IV and VIII

(5) To pass on to ख or आकाश *i. e.* ether. "We assume that there is a medium between the earth and the sun and stars distinct from ordinary matter. This medium is called the luminous ether, or simply the ether, sometimes spelt aether to distinguish it from the ether that can be bought at a chemist's shop in bottles. The aether has no weight (it must have some weight but it is inappreciable by our senses)* it fills all space of matter." (Houstoun)

Modern science proves that the material world is in incessant motion and is composed of ether.

This ether is called आकाश *Akash.* It is not vacuum as ignorantly believed or supposed by some but an element which is present in everything in this universe, and in which this earth and all the heavenly bodies float. There is no vacuum in this universe as the whole myriad of space is occupied by ether.

---

* It is the primeval element or primordeal substance from which this whole universe is evolved.

"The three physical states in which matter exists are called gaseous, liquid and solid and differ from each other not in actual structure but in degrees of compression."

All substances, without exception, are regarded by science as made up of extremely small particles called "Molecules." Molecules are made up of smaller particles called "atoms". and Atoms are made up of still smaller particles called "electrones" (ions). Every molecule is in a constant state of rapid motion or oscillation and is quite separated from every other molecule. However small the distance between the molecules no amount of pressure can drive one into another. The spaces between the molecules of all substances which we are able to see, feel, weigh, etc. with our ordinary senses are occupied by some invisible substance. This substance is called "ether". It is present every-where between the molecules of all solids, liquids and gases and fills all the "*void*" between the earth, planets and stars. Through this elther the planets move in space round the Sun and through it the molecules of substances are always journeying to and fro.

There are several varieties of ether :—

1. The Thermal Ether (Red ether) constitutes the ordinary coarser grades of heat.

2. The Thermo—Lumino-Ether is the orange ether which is visible in **गोमेदस** orange coloured precious stone and yellowish tinted diamond.

(3) Electro-Ether is blue coloured ether, it is the element of frictional electricity. Dr. Babbitt says it is more electrical than the other elements of electricity.

(4) Electro-lumino Ether is of blue green colour. These colour-ethers grow finer as they progress through thermal red, red orange, orange, etc., up to dark violet and really far beyond that although they become invisible to the ordinary eye (Babbitt.) So also there exist Chemico ether, Galvano ether, Magneto ether Odylo ether, Psychic ether, Psycho ether, Gravite ether, Cosmic ether, etc.

"These different ethers play an important part in heat, light, electricity, magnetism, etc. Our very thoughts and feelings being a part of the cosmos are composed of vibrations of ether. An act of our will is composed of etheric vibrations. It must necessarily set in motion a certain amount of etheric energy; the stronger the will the greater the amount of energy it commands" (Lovel).

Dr. Lindlahr says "we can by the power of will direct the vital currents to those parts and organs which need them most and we can relieve congested areas by equalizing the circulation by drawing therefrom the surplus of blood and nerve currents and distributing the vital fluids over other parts of the body."

Thus by the power of will we can control not only the vital functions in our own bodies but also in other persons as mesmerists and hypnotists do. Hindu Yogis develop this power to a marvellous extent.

Hindu Yogis have a wide spread reputation of their ability to cure all sorts of nervous diseases. They sprinkle some water, apply some ashes, or recite some incantations by holding their right hand on the patient's head or heart, A young woman aged 20 years was on the point of death on account of difficult labour; the attending midwife was entirely helpless. She suggested surgeon's interference. A Yogi with a few passes and suggestions not only alleviated all her pangs but also caused an easy delivery.

A young boy aged 14 years had an injury which turned into an obstinate indolent ulcer; an Ayurvedic physician and an Allopathic doctor failed to cure it. The Doctor suggested operation. But a few compresses of pure water prepared by adding a little ash given by a Yogi almost cured it. Later on a little cow's ghee supplied by the same Yogi after reciting some incantations cured the ulcer completely.

A theft of an ornament took place in a house during the marriage ceremony of the occupant's daughter. He did not report the matter to the police but consulted a Yogi who asked him to call on him with a boy or a girl aged about 10 years in the evening. Accordingly the gentleman went to him with his friend's niece aged nine. She was then bathed and made to sit down in a room containing a dim cocoanut oil lamp. The Yogi then brought a betel leaf, made a small circular mark over it of cows ghee and made that girl to gaze over it sitting near the lamp. After a few minutes he suggested to her that she would be able to see the ornament, belonging to so and so which was stolen on a particular day; she gave the description of that ornament and said that it was kept in his box by the owner (giving the description and not the name) at such and such a time. He asked "Is it still there or removed and if removed how ? and by whom ? She said "A young man whose age is so much whose features are such and such and whose dress is such and such removed it with the help of a duplicate key. He "asked what has he done with it ? She replied "He has buried it under a mango tree on the southern side." He asked. "Is it still there ? She replied" "yes". The gentleman went there with an honest servant and a spade and found the ornament there in tact.

A gentleman lost 5 currency notes worth Rupees 100 each kept in his box. Then a young boy of ten years was hypnotised; he said a man whose age is so much whose features are such and who wears such dress has removed them with the help of a duplicate key and has now kept them in such a house, such a room and in such a box in the left side compartment in an envelope which bears such superscription. He also gave the numbers of those notes in that hypnotic trance. When the person was threatened with the help of a police man he expressed regret and made over the notes to the person concerned with a profuse apology.

Convulsions and Hysteria:—The author has cured over a dozen obstinate cases of convulsions of infants, with mesmeric passes and half a dozen cases of obstinate hysteria with mesmeric passes and suggestions.

Sleeplessness:—A young girl aged 17 years had no sleep for over two weeks and had become very irritable. Her parents were naturally anxious and feared that she might go mad. At the author's visit he found her lying as usual in an arm chair with her eyes wide open (at 10-30 P.M.). He made some passes with his left hand by making her hold fast two of his fingers of the right hand with her both hands and suggested that she would soon feel sleepy and sleep till next morning undisturbed. To the surprise of her relations the suggestion came true. To cure her of sleeplessness entirely she had to be mesmerised seven times on aternate days and given suggestions as follows "you will be all right and your sleeplessness will disappear entirely in two weeks; keep your mind cool and remember these my words whenever you don't feel sleepy"

Sleeplessness :—A woman aged 27 was sleepless both during night and day; she had taken opium, bromide, chloral hydrate, etc. under Ayurvedic and Allopathic treatment; she suffered for three months. She used to get a short sleep as the effect of these drugs with tired feeling nextday; but never otherwise. When on a visit in the neighbourhood the author was asked to examine and treat her; he made her hold two fingers of his right hand with both her hands one finger with each hand and made some mesmeric passes suggesting that she would not feel sleepy then, but feel so at 10 the very night. These suggestions had very satisfactory result, she did get sleep at 10 p. m. She needed to be mesmerised twenty one times in the same way before she was able to overcome her sleeplessness completely.

Abscess :—An Allopathic doctor friend of the author once took him to the former's patient whose heart was weak and who was suffering from a painful abscess on her right breast which he wanted to cut open. The author made some mesmeric passes and *suggested* that she would not feel pain while cutting it open and while dressing it. She was lively and did not show any signs of pain to the surprise of the doctor and her relatives.

Toothache :—A young lady in a village was suffering from terrible tooth-ache which did not yield to fomentations, cloves, camphor, etc. At 10–30 P. M. the author made some passes and suggested that all her suffering would be mitigated on account of the passes he had made. Soon she felt relieved of her pain and was able to sleep till the next morning. In the morning when she got up she felt no tooth ache.

Entertainment :—The author had an occasion to mesmerise a boy aged 12, at the request of an elderly relative curious to witness mesmerism of which he had heard so much. The boy was made to hold fast two fingers of the right hand of the author who then made some passes with his left hand; the boy soon entered the hypnotic trance. When asked to dash his head against the wall after some passes on the head and suggestions that he would not feel pain he did so but showed no signs of pain. Again, after some passes on his left thigh, he was asked to prick his thigh with a needle where the author made passes with an assurance that no blood or pain would result, he did so and all those who were present there witnessed the scene; the boy showed no signs of pain and no blood came out of

11

his thigh. A pot of boiling water was brought and kept there and the boy was asked to dip his right hand fingers in it, the author suggested to him that the water would not be hot to the touch, he was able to keep his fingers under the water until the author asked him to remove them from boiling water; the fingers had no blisters nor did they look reddish. A box was brought and kept before the boy the contents of which he did not know But when asked by the author what were the contents of the box he gave detailed list of its contents with full description to the satisfaction and surprise of all who had gathered there.

The mind is to the body as force to Matter.

THE MIND

The mind has three aspects (1) सत्वगुण the intellect, (2) रजोगुण the will and तमोगुण the emotions.

(1) The Intellect सत्वगुण Satwaguna.

The intellect enables us to distinguish good from bad, to solve difficult problems, to think, guess and predict right things, etc. Aryabhat's statement that the Earth was turning round the sun made 2200 years ago, Caxton's invention of the art of printing, Lesseps' project of Suez canal, Newton's discovery of the Law of gravitation, and Hahnemann's application of the Law of Similars to the art of healing are all the works of intelligence. They all were intellectual giants.

(2) **The Will** रजोगुण Rajoguna.

The will gives the power to do or undo certain things and aspire higher things. The grandest object of the will if it is not corrupted is always good; and our great object should always be to cultivate it and develop it to its highest capacity and not to misdirect it or corrupt it in any way. Emerson says "The one serious and formidable thing in Nature is our will". In good old times Krishna wanted to exterminate all wicked persons from this Earth. Though he was not powerful himself to do so, with his astute statesmanship he was able to do so after all. Ashoka determined to spread Buddhism as much as possible and he was able to do so, not only in India and Ceylon but in the whole of Asia. Alexander the great determined to conquer the whole known world and he was able to do so. Shankar the illustrious commentator of *Brahma-sutras* and *Bhagavadgita* determined to turn a *Sanyasee* and establish monasteries to spread *Adwaita* philosophy. There were so many obstacles in his way. He being the only male child in the family and being fatherless he could not obtain the permission of his mother who wanted to get him married and according to the rules of the *Sanyasees* he could not turn a Sanyasee without the consent of his mother. At last she was forced to give her consent as he was bent upon turning a sanyasee and luckily he got an able (Guru) teacher who taught him Sanskrit and Vedant philosophy. He established five monasteries which are still conducted in his name. He is now known all over the world and his name has become immortal. Some even deify him. Ramadas, a Sanyasee and a beggar saw the spread of Mohamedan power and religion in the Deccan under the powerful Mogul Emperor Aurangzeb and determined to establish a Hindu kingdom to prevent Hindus and cows being killed. He succeeded remarkably with the help of *Shivaji* who risked his own life several times and established a Hindu kingdom according to the desire of his *guru.* Shivaji is now deified. Those who have read the life of Napoleon know of his great achievements.

These examples illustrate the capabilities of will power or determination.

(3) The Emotion तमोगुण Tamoguna.

Emotion is the sudden excitement or agitation of mind, when a person decides on a certain course of action. For instance Gautama Buddha got up in the dead of night and suddenly decided to eschew his kingly state, his throne, his beloved wife and his new born babe and retire to the forest in search of means of release from earthly bondage and suffering. Bhartrihari in a fit of dispair deserted his throne and repaired to the forest, where he lived as an ascetic though he had the power to punish his wife whom he suspected of unfaithfulness and wed another. Sudden desire felt in the mind for a strange woman, sudden inclination to wound the feelings of others and sudden thought to commit homicide or suicide in certain persons are also mental emotions or तमोगुण aspects of mind.

Hindu sages of old have divided our food stuffs into three classes. सात्विक *satwik* developing Intellect राजस *Rajus* developing Will power and तामस *Tamus* developing Emotions. According to them all fruits, nuts, roots, leaves, flowers, and vegetables except onion and garlic, milk, curds, buttermilk, sugar-cane and grains such as rice, wheat, millet, maize, oats, etc. are *satwik* foodstuffs. All pulses, potatoes, sweet potatoes, all cooked food stuff's from so many roots and starchy substances having sweet, sour, saltish and astringent taste are *Rajus* food-stuffs, while flesh-meat, fish, fowl, pickles, *chutnees*, *papads* and other pungent things, onion, garlic, cloves, cinnamon, ginger and other heaty food, all intoxicating drinks, coffee, tobaccc, opium and other narcotics, tea, wines, beer and other stimulating drinks, all cooked food with sea-salt, chillies, mustard, spices, etc. are *Tamas* food stuffs. It is well known that those who eat more of fruits and nuts are thin, enduring and very intelligent and are also calm and quiet and those who take *Rajas* food, are fat, ambitious and men of strong determinations while flesh meat-eaters, drunkards, smokers and coffee drinkers, as a rule are of excitable temper and cruel.

Psycho-therapy or Mind-cure.

Our body is controlled by our mind, while our mind is inspired by our consciousness, an attribute of our soul which is a part and parcel of the universal soul. There is no doubt that we can control the diseases both of body and mind by giving hopes and assurances to the patient. There are some who can fill others with hope and cheer and others who can not. An experienced nurse very often soothes the mind and relieves the sufferings of her patient. An experienced Ayurvedic physician very often quotes a suitable Sanskrit verse from the old authors and explains its meaning to his patient saying that a certain drug is an excellent remedy for his malady as some kind of humour is in excess in his body; then the patient feels cheered and confident of his cure, so that he feels considerably relieved in mind.

A patient very often feels that he is almost cured when a cheerful nurse assures him that she has seen worse cases cured and he would get all right in a very short time.

A student of the author who is now practising in Homoeopathy and Biochemistry told him that the verses composed by the author on Homoeopathic and Biochemic Materia Medica have been of great use to him, as he cited some to three of his patients with the result that he inspired them with confidence and hope and they felt half cured of their maladies.

Dr. Lindlahr says—"Every thought and every emotion has its direct effect upon the physical constituents of the body. The mental and emotional vibrations become physical vibrations and structures. Discord in the mind is translated into disease in the body while the harmonies of hope, faith, cheerfulness, happiness, love and altruism create in the organism the corresponding health vibrations".

In *Vedant* philosophy it is said that we have in this our स्थूलदेह physical body, one सूक्ष्मदेह astral (ethereal) body which governs our mind; our will-power is dependent on it. First we must strengthen the will, then we must direct it towards what is good by fixing the mind on it and meditating on it. We should not expect nor attempt for too much in the beginning. The success in spreading religious beliefs is based on the perseverence and steadiness of the founders and those who attempted to spread them.

Forgetfulness and idleness are the enemies of our will, we should try to cultivate the memory by concentrating our will with etheric power and by-the-by success will be ours. It is now a well-known fact that though suggestions or psycho-therapy is not itself able to cure all diseases, it helps a good deal to cure many of them chiefly nervous disorders and mental troubles.

" There are various terms " says Lowel " with which most people are familiar such as Faith-cure, Christian Science-cure, Mental healing, Will-cure, Hypnotic suggestion, Curative mesmerism, etc. The basis of all these is etheric vibration influenced by the will of the person himself or of another for it is a demonstrated fact that the ether penetrates every material substance without exception; an act of will being composed of etheric vibratary energy.

The following quotation from the Herald of Health April 1919 will show that the attempt of some persons to cure all diseases only with faith or suggestions is merely ridiculous.

Query : " Hallow John ! I hear your father was cured of rheumatism by Christian science "

Reply : " Oh no, he was cured of Christian science by rheumatism ".

Rheumatism, gout, migraine, neuralgia, sciatica, sprue, diarrhoea, dysentery, cholera, boils, abscesses, carbuncles, cancers, etc. cannot be cured by faith or suggestions alone; they need sunlight, water, diet, and sometimes suitable homoeopathic medicines also which work according to the Law of Similars. Dr. Lindlahr and others also hold the same opinion.

Electricity.

Since the discovery of electricity the scientist and the physician have been incessantly at work to harness it to the best advantage in their individual field of effort. The scientist prepared machines called Static, Faradic, Galvanic, etc. of different strength and some physicians undertook to treat with electricity patients who had been disappointed with medicine; even such of them as felt slightly better after the current had been applied, grew worse on account of the after effects produced by the strong currents generated by the batteries employed; so also indiscrete use of electricity is also harmful. The human body also has negative and positive poles (see Plate No. 1.). To slacken the stiff parts apply positive Electricity to the negative parts and negative Electricity to the positive parts and to stiffen the slack muscles apply positive to the positive and negative to the negative. (See Electro-Homeopathy by the author.) Count Caesar Mattei was the first to denounce the method of applying strong electricity He also prepared some negative and positive feeble liquid electricities from plants only; they produced better results than the strong currents generated from metals. In 1900 Nickola Tesla realised that in the human system vibration was the greatest factor and that the sense of hearing, smelling and seeing were due to vibration of the ether ; he also observed that these senses responded in proportion to the number of vibrations that were received per minute. Therefore, he maintains that if electricity is to be applied to the human system it should be very feeble *i. e.* in an acceptable form to harmonize the system by raising the vibrations in the body. He thus increased the vibrations to 40,000 per minute and reduced the amperage to almost nothing in his Violet Ray machine. Violet and ultra-violet rays obtained from the sun on high mounts have the better effects in healing any disease chiefly rickets, phthisis and tuberculosis of any variety, because they are natural. Unscrupulous manufacturers have been preparing Violet Ray machines not in accordance with this principles. Hence such machines are not able to yield benefical results while natural sun baths and water baths with appropriate massage (see chapter X) produce satisfactory results.

Magnetism

We have different forms of magnetism such as :— metal magnetism, vegetable magnetism and animal magnetism. Metal magnetism is fully dealt with in every treatise on magnetism;–vegetable or plant magnetism also repel similar and attract dissimilar magnetism of its kind; animal or human magnetism has also attracting and repelling properties. Those who have developed this power can, not onlv heal diseases but even fascinate living beings. Not only human beings but even cattle and serpents are magnetised and fascinated by them in a wonderful manner.

Animal Magnetism

From time immemorial Hindoos, Greeks, Romans, Arabs, Hebrews, Assyrians, Jews, Chinese, Japanese and other nations were making use of animal magnetism in the art of healing and some of them still do it.

Animal magnetism is the name used to describe the subtle sympathetic life-force by which certain persons are able to influence, attract and even cure other persons. If their influence is good they are said to impart "a heallthy magnetism. Mesmerism is a term of similar import, and was given to the practice of Animal Magnetism by the followers of Mesmer. Hypnotism is a more modern term originally suggested and employed by Dr. Braid of Manchester and for all practical purposes is synonymous to the forgoing (Cotes).

Mesmerism.

" Mesmer, having learnt the art of curing disease (with animal magnetism) from Father Hehl applied himself to the cure of disease with "extraordinary success." He left Viena, and travelling through out Germany and Switzerland, he continued to work wonder; his cures approximating to the miraculous. Kings and courtiers as well as the people vied with one another for an opportunity to attend his *Levees* and partake in his *Seances*. In 1778 he started for Paris; here his success in curing disease was so remarkable that the elite of society struggled for the privilege of waiting upon him and of learning his art. A society was actually formed for the purpose of acquiring his secret and using it for the cure of disease ". (Cotes).

Human Aura

" About the middle of the nineteenth century Baron von Reichenbach, a German scientist, took up the work where Mesmer had left it and brought actual proof of the existence of the electro-magnetic energies and of their manifestation in the aura. He conducted his experiments in a dark chamber impervious to light rays from outside. Psychically sensitive persons after remaining in his dark chamber for a short time, were able to perceive the aura more or less distinctly in the form of light or bluish vapour emanating from living objects placed before them. Clairvoyant Psychics or sensitives, as he called them, were able to distinguish various colours of the aura. " (Lindlahr)

"The following simple experiment will make the purely physical emanations of the aura visible to ordinary sight in a room dark enough to leave the hands just visible, alternately approach and separate the finger tips. If a person is in good, healthy physical condition streaks of bluish light or vapour will appear between the finger tips "

Magnetic Treatment

" The principal rule to be obsesved by the physician when administering magnetic treatment is to place himself in such a position to the subject that opposite parts of their bodies come into juxtaposition, that is the right hand must touch or pass over the left side of the patient, and vice versa."

"When giving the magnetic passes in a sitting position the subject should remain in a comfortable, relaxed and receptive condition. The more receptive and sensitive the subject, the more distinctly he will feel the magnetic vibrations like a mild current from an electric battery."

"Magnetic passes must proceed from the head down-ward over the body, the hands returning in a sweeping out-ward, circular movement so as not to counteract the down-ward passes"

Positive and Negative Magnetism

"Water may be charged with positive or negative magnetism as required by the character of the ailment; positeve magntism has an astringent effect upon the tissues of the body, while negative magnetism has a relaxing effect. Positive magnetism, therefore, would be in order for the treatment of chronic diarrhoea, while negative magnetism is most effective for the treatment of constipation."

"In order to charge water or any other fluid positively the left hand is placed under the vessel, while the right hand with fingers pointing down-ward and in close proximity to the fluid makes circular passes. If a substance is to be magnetised negatively, the process would he reversed, that is the fingers of the left hand must do the charging. In like manner, fabrics and other substances may be charged magnetically." (Lindlahr)

The followers of Mesmer believe in animal magnetism, they say one can develop it in one's own self and can make use of it in entertainments and curing diseases by imparting it through passes to any other person. With these passes not only several obstinate nervous diseases can be cured but also surgical operations can he performed without causing any pain to the patients. During entertainments the skin of the healthy persons can he made insensible to such an extent that needles can be poked in it without causing bleeding or pain to the person.

Hypnotism.

In 1842 Dr. Braid taught that the hypnotic condition could be induced without mesmeric passes or without the intervention of a second person by means of concentration of the gaze upon a bright object. This method of hynotising persons is very common in Southern India from time immemorial. A piece of glass or a beetle leaf with a round mark of cows ghee or oil is placed near a dim light and any person is asked to see it carefully and concentrate his mind and sight over it. The person soon gets sleepy and in that hypnotic state he sees all what is required in that glass or the round shining mark made over the leaf by the hypnotiser. Not only can thefts be detected in this way but also certain events happening in other countries read. A hypnotised person can even tell what is kept in a locked cupboard or box.

"I have seen a weak young woman under the control of a hypnotist display sufficient physical energy to overcome the concentrated efforts of four strong men

.o lift her from the floor or to move her from her place. I have seen her lift weight which could not be raised by two or three strong men. On another occasion I saw a weak boy carry the hypnotist, a man weighing over a hundred and seventy pounds, on his outstretched, unsupported arm. The hypnotist in these cases was not reinforcing his subjects by his own muscular strength. Their greatly increased physical strength and stamina were entirely due to the power of will, acting on their subconscious minds through hypnotic control". (Lindlahr)

During such mesmeric influence and hypnotic ate, through suggestions not only can pains be itigated but also diseases cured in a wonderful manner. Dr. Rutland states there is no disease physical or functional that is accompanied by discomfort or pain which may not be relieved to some extent by suggestions given during hypnotic state.

" Amongst the striking cases with which I have dealt I may mention a girl of twentyhree who had suffered from epileptic fits for years. She had consumed so much bromide" during her childhood that she had a permanent rash on her forehead which quite disfigured her. I hypnotised her regularly each week for six months and the interverls between the attacks gradually increased where as the severity of the seizures diminished. This improvement was maintained and the face rash disappearing she was revealed as a good-looking girl and when I last heard of her was engaged to be married" (Dr. Rutland).

At the age of seventy a Scottish lady fell ill and her disease was diagnosed as incurable and multiple abdominal cancer; she had a horror of the surgeon's knife and she even shrank from the idea of a hypodermic injection of morphia; but by means of suggestion I was able to mitigate her sufferings and her last words were to the effict that she was comfortable and free from pain. During my absence abroad a few weeks before her death, a medical friend looked after her on my behalf, and administered frequent doses of morphia and other anodynes, but failed to relieve the incessant pain (Rutland).

So rapid a spread of Theosophy in India, the land of *yogis* and philosophers was partly due to some of the wonderful cures effected by Col. Olcott with hypnotic and mesmeric powers. Rutland states "he once hypnotised a wounded man and made him forget all but his fatal injuries and cured them in an incredibly short period. He could even order and give instructions to his body-servant by Telepathy without the use of speech and at any distance".

"Telepathy is the transmission of thoughts from mind to mind through vibrations in the ether. If it is possible for metal instruments to transmit messages through thousands of miles of open wireless space, why should it be impossible to send mental vibrations from mind to mind and brain to brain through the all-pervading ether? A few years ago materialistic science would have dismissed telepathy as another evidence of hysterical self delusion or as tricks of pretenders and *fakirs*". (Lindlahr).

CHAPTER VIII.

Breathing Exercise, General and Psychic; Fresh Air and Proper Breathing.

"Good air is an important element in a natural way of living and healing" (Platen).

If pure blood is the sustainer of life—fresh air is the purifier and supporter of blood; not only do both our lungs but also all our pores inhale fresh air constantly and supply oxygen to our blood if we allow them to do so. Therefore it is very necessary that we should spend as much of our days and nights as possible in fresh air only. A human being is an air animal; he needs continuously fresh air for his skin as much as for the inner side of his lungs. Without food and water an animal can live for some time; but without air it can not live even for a few minutes. In impure air a man will die or will find his health impaired. Hence it is very necessary that we should always live in and continuously breathe pure air. Impure air can not be made worth-inhaling by perfumes, scents, otto of roses, Eu de cologne or by fumigation with odorous substances as they will make the air further unfit for inhalation; Nature wants us to inhale pure air, rich with oxygen, the life-supporting element.

Kind Nature has supplied us with pure air bountifully; but where shall we breathe it? If we go to public roads there the air is contaminated with offensive smell of the tar which is spread all over the roads for the facility of the motor car drivers and the felicity of the motor car owners. Offensive gases are often ejected from their motors. Restaurants are full of the strong odour of spices and of vapours produced by frying which excites terrible cough. Public buildings, lecture halls, theatres, workshops, colleges and schools are full of effluvia aud tobacco smoke. Public gardens are filled with smoke and dust proceeding from flour mills and cotton mills and railway engines. Even in the so called non-smoking compartments of the railway trains, we get the smoke blown on us; there too we are oppressed by the smoke of tobacco and sparks of fire coming from smoking compartments, which often burn our clothes. Old persons, young men and tender boys and even budding young women are seen smoking and offering cigars and cigarettes to their friends and the atmosphere surrounding them is found full of nicotine poison and the gas produced from igniting matches.

Pet monkeys have been seen smoking cigars with gusto. Boys either offer us a cigar or ask us to give one to them or claim matches from us to light their cigars; and if we tell them that we do not smoke, they do not believe us, as they are under the impression that smoking is an essential need of human beings. Our public buildings have become nicotine dens. Almost every building on the high road possesses one country tobacco-shop and more than one shop selling European cigars. No restaurant is considered up-to-date unless it can supply costly cigars. Some allopathic doctors recommend smoking for dyspepsia and flatulence instead of recommending some exercise or a change in diet.

Some *Unanee Hakeems* prepare a special scented tobacco for chewing and smoking with the addition of musk, amber, and other substances which cause sexual excitement in the beginning and sexual weakness and depression, nervousness, scurvy, pyorrhoea, etc. later on. Without knowing its after-effects many rich persons make use of it freely and suffer from its consequences. There is no wonder, therefore, that the percentages of illness and mortality are higher in towns than they are in villages. At this rate the atmosphere in towns will, in course of time, get so much contaminated as to become unfit for the inhalation of human beings and with a little exaggeration, we may say, that it may cause suffocation even to the birds of the air from the smoke we emit from this globe.

It will be interesting to find how the most eminent modern writers on hygiene agree with the most ancient medical writer *Charaka* regarding the use of pure air. See chapter 1 Regarding Charak's views. (1) " Health is only possible when to other conditions is added that of a proper supply of pure air." (2) " Air is the prime supporter of life and health, even life itself is dependent upon its purity." (3) Statistical inquiries on mortality prove beyond a doubt that of the causes of death which are usually in action, impurity of the air is the most important. (Parkes)

" Inhale slowly, always through the nostrils prolonging the act as much as possible and filling the lungs, the lower as well as the upper parts with air; then give less time to exhaling and let every exhalation be forcible and accompanied by an abdominal movement which will aid in emptying the stagnant cells in the lower part of the lungs" (Hunter) See pages 186 and 187.

General Breathing Exercises.

I. *Breathing for Heart and Lung Stimulation*

(1) Stand erect facing the sun with hands at sides.

(2) Breathe in slowly and steadily

(3) While breathing gently tap the chest with your finger tips

(4) When the lungs are full retain the breath and rub the chest with your own palms.

II. *Breathing for Rib-strengthening*

(1) Stand erect facing the sun with palms touching the ribs.

(2) Inhale a complete breath slowly.

(3) Retain the inhaled air for a short time.

(4) Rub your Ribs gently with your palms while exhaling.

III. *Breathing for Expansion of Chest.*

(1) Stand erect facing the sun extending both arms forward on a level with the shoulders

(2) Inhale a complete breath till chest is full

(3) Retain the air as long as possible and stretch the arms sideways straight with the shoulders.

(4) Then exhale rubbing the chest forcibly with your own palms.

IV. *Breathing Exercise for Preserving Health.*

(1) Stand erect facing the sun, stretch both hands at sides, inhale deeply and exhale slowly; then raise the arms up until palms touch each other and rise up on the toes as high as possible. Inhale while rising up and raising hands and exhale while lowering the heels and hands slowly and steadily.

(2) Stand erect facing the sun, rub the chest with your right palm and inhale deeply; then exhale slowly and while exhaling clap the chest with both the palms.

V. *Breathing Exercise for the Sick and the Invalids to Recoup Health.*

(1) Lie on your back on the ground well cleaned for this purpose or on a carpet; stretch your head towards the north pole and your hands above the head and raise your knees. Then breathe deeply and steadily several times. While inhaling raise the abdomen as high as possible and draw it in as deep as possible while exhaling.

(2) Lie on your back and stretch both the hands on both sides. Inhale slowly and deeply filling in and emptying the lungs freely. Do this several times. Then turn to the left side and do the same, then turn to the right side and do the same.

Natural Breathing

Deep breathing is natural and entirely involuntary among those who do not overload the stomach or do obey Nature's demands. It is one of the organic functions carried on by bodily forces entirely independent of the lung activity. It purifies the blood, strengthens the heart with the oxygen inhaled, quickens the circulation of blood, distributes highly oxygenated vitalizing blood all over the body, increases the vitality and establishes immunity from disease.

Correct breathing supplies more oxygen to the blood, circulates it properly and purifies it, which can be clearly observed by clear and bright complexion, while the blood of those who breathe imperfectly is bluish, darkish, and lacking in oxygen which can be observed by livid or pale complexion.

Proper breathing not only improves one's health but also mental powers, and clearsightedness. It also enables one to have a control ovor the passions and insures immunity from disease.

The air on the sea-shore contains, ·090 percent more oxygen than the air of the town. While the air in the town contains about 0·05 percent of carbonic acid, the air on lofty mountains contains more of oxygen and carbonic acid and less of organic matter than the air in districts while the atmosphere of the town contains diminished proportion of oxygen.

"A proper supply of pure fresh air" says Dr. Ruddock "is essential to the preservation and enjoyment of life and health, by breathing an impure atmosphere the vital energies are slowly but surely impaired".

Air loaded with effluvia" says Bernan "from the lungs, skin, and clothes even of a healthy individual is offensive to a certain extent, but from that of a person in a state of disease prevented by the walls and ceiling from escaping is in the highest degree deleterious and loathsome".

Psychical Breathing Exercises.

प्राणवायु *Pranavayu* or oxygen enters the body chiefly through the nostrils and also through the pores. Hence the necessity of exposing the whole skin to pure fresh air and bright sunlight and also inhaling the air through the nostrils and not through the mouth. The breath taken through the left nostril creates negative electromagnetic currents on the left side of the body, while the breath taken through the right nostril creates positive electromagnetic currents on the right side of the body.

If a person has got the faulty habit of breathing through the mouth or if he suffers from frequent attacks of catarrh, polypus, formation of crusts, etc. the right method of breathing may be established and other troubles cured by practising psychical breathing exercises preseribed in the Yoga philosophy under the heading of Pranayama.

These breathing exercises keep the blood pure and bring the individual human soul in intimate connection with the universal soul, the great reservoir of life without which life would be extinct.

Atma or soul is the real self. It is not the body nor the mind of man. The body and the mind are but parts of his personality. Atma is the ego or the real self. It is independent of the body which it inhabits and the mind is its instrument to do all actions good or bad. The real self or *Jeevatma* is an atom of the universal soul or *Paramatma*. It is eternal and immortal. It is also indestructible. It does not die nor can it be annihilated nor changed in its form like those ingredients of the body. The ingredients of the body are also indestructible; they are developed to the present state from the crude ingredients of the universe or Brahma. They are undergoing changes every day and change entirely when the soul abandons them. They are also formed from ingredients which can neither be created nor destroyed.

By practising Pranayama mentioned in Yoga and meditation one can realise the existence of the soul and the idea of yourself being the soul and its condition independent of the body.

Psychical Breathing Exercises According to the *Yoga* Philosophy.

अथातः संप्रवक्ष्यामि प्राणायामस्य सद्विधिम् ।
यस्य साधनमात्रेण चिरंजीवी भवेन्नरः ॥ १ ॥

Translation—I now narate the methods of *Pranayama* or Breathing Exercise which, if practised properly will prolong life.

यावद् वायुःस्थितो देहे तावज् जीवनमुच्यते ।
मरणं तस्य निष्क्रान्ति रततो वायुं निरोधयेत् ॥ २ ॥

Translation–Man remains alive so long as he can breathe; he ceases to live as soon as he ceases to breathe.

Therefore one should know fully well how to exercise one's breath.

हिताहारं मिताहारं नाडीशुद्धिंतथैवच ।
तत्पश्चान्मनसः शान्ति प्राणायामंच साधयेत् ॥ ३ ॥

Translation–One should take only wholesome food in moderation and keep one's body clean, (with baths and by removing constipation). After that one should keep one's mind contented and then practise *Pranayama*.

शरीरलाघवं सम्यगुत्साहो मनसस्तथा ।
अरोगताच तेजश्च लभ्यन्ते नाडिशोधनात् ॥ ४ ॥

Translation–Leanness of the body, energy of mind, good health and brilliance are obtained by keeping the body pure and free from impurities.

स-कारेण विशत्यंतर् यात्यऽहं-कारतो बाहिः ।
सोऽहमित्यव्ययं मंत्रं जीवो जपति सर्वदा ॥ ५॥

Translation—The *Pranavayu* enters the body with the sound स *sa* and goes out with the sound अहं *Aham*; thus the life force always recites the मन्त्र—सोऽहम् *soham* incantation always.

सोऽहम् means *I am He i. e.* the life soul is the universal (and no other) soul.

According to its position in the body the wind is named प्राण Prana, अपान Apana, व्यान Vyana, उदान Udana and समान Samana.

हृदि प्राणो गुदेऽपानः समानो नाभिसंस्थितः ।
उदानः कण्ठदेशेच व्यानः सर्वशरीरगः ॥ ६ ॥

(1) *Pranavayu* occupies the lungs in the region of the chest; it is the bodily vital activity.

(2) *Apana vayu* occupies the lower bowel and governs the excretory functions.

(3) *Vyana vayu* pervades the whole body and holds itself fast in all its parts.

(4) *Udana* is the ascending vayu or the so called upward breathing; its usual position is the region of larynx.

(5) *Samana vayu* occupies the abdominal region and governs the digestive functions and assimilation of food and keeps up the normal heat of the body with the hedp of तेज *Tej* element.

Pranayama or Psychic Breathing Exercise for preserving health and prolnging life.

General Rules.

(A) Pranayama should not be practised :—

(1) when one is hungry or thirsty or tired

(2) when the stomach is full. (A Yogi should not overload the stomach.)

(3) when the mind is not at ease.

(4) when one is ill or angry (as a rule a Yogi does not get ill or excited.)

(5) where there is offensive smell or where some artificial odours are spread such as of camphor, sulphur, phenyle, iodo-form, etc. or where there is smoke or dust.

(B) It should be performed :—

(1) In the morning, noon, evening or at bedtime

(2) In well-ventilated rooms or halls.

(3) On the banks of rivers on the sea-shore or on the slopes of mounts containing air rich with oxygen

(4) Under a Bael tree, a Neem tree, a Banian tree or a Peepal tree as these give out oxygen and purify the surrounding air

(5) In a garden, in the bright sun, or near a tree or creeper bearing fragrant flowers or near Tulsi plants which purify the surrounding air.

प्राणःस्वदेहजो वायुरायाम स्तन्निरोधनम् ।
प्राणायामँस्त्रिधा प्रोक्तः पूरकुम्भकरेचकैः ॥ ७ ॥

Translation :—That original life-breath in our body which dwells in the region of our chest is called *Prana* or life. *Ayama* is its exercise. Exercising the breath properly and spreading it all over the chest is called *Pranayama*. It is of three sorts *pooraka*, *Kumbhaka* and *Rechaka*.

बाह्यादापूरणं वायो रुदरे पूरकः स्मृतः ।
संपूर्णं कुम्भवत्तस्य धारणं कुंभको भवेत् ॥ ८ ॥

तद् वायो रेचनं बाह्य रेचकं कथ्यते बुधैः ।
प्राणायामेन युक्तेन सर्व रोगक्षयो भवेत् ॥ ९ ॥

Translation :—Inhalation of the air is called Pooraka ; holding in the lungs the inhaled air is called Kumbhaka ; and the exhalation of the inhaled air is called Rechaka by wise Yogis. By practising these proper methods of pranayama one can cure all diseases.

इडा वामे स्थिता नाडी पिंगला दक्षिणे तथा।
सुषुम्ना मध्यदेशे च प्रोक्ता योगविशारदैः ॥ १० ॥

Expert Yogis have demonstrated that the *Ida* nerve exists in the left and *Pingala* nerve in the right side of our body while *Sushumna* nerve is in the middle of our body.

पूरकांते कुंभकांतं धार्यं नासापुटद्वयम् ।
कनिष्ठानामिकांगुष्ठै स्तर्जनीं मध्यमांविना ॥ ११ ॥

(1) Exhale first thoroughly by holding the spine, neck and head straight; then try *pooraka* by *Ida i. e.* close the right nostril first and inhale through the left fully; then observe *Kumbhaka*, i. e. hold the air in the lungs by closing both the nostrils right with the right thumb and left with the shortest finger of the right hand and the finger near it; and then do *Rechaka i. e.* exhale slowly all the air through the right nostril by closing the left one. As the heart is on the left side of the chest the left lung must be oxidised first to strengthen the heart and purify the blood. Then close the left nostril and inhale through the right one; hold the air in as long as possible and then exhale it slowly through the left nostril. Repeat these processes six to ten times thrice a day. Once in the morning standing near an open window, then at noon sitting or standing in the bright sun and lastly at night in bed in a lying position; the windows of the room must always be kept open to admit fresh air.

This sort of morning breathing exercese is good for preserving health, the noon exercise is useful in healing diseases and the night exercise is helpful in inducing a quiet and refreshing sleep.

(2) Inhale by the right nostril and exhale by the left 10 to 16 times; do so thrice daily morning, noon and evening. This method is called *Sooryabhedana*. It cures liver troubles and brightens the features.

(3) Attain a straight position and inhale through both nostrils by closing the mouth properly; hold the breath as long as possible and then exhale as slowly as possible. This method is called *Bhramaree* and is useful to purify the blood; it keeps the mind calm and quiet, and produces a pleasant sensation after the exercise and is very useful for the preservation of health.

(4) Close the mouth and inhale fresh air through both the nostrils slowly and steadily ; then have a long pause to retain the inhaled air and extend the chest walls and expand the lungs as much as possible ; and then expel slowly through the left nostril. This breathing exercise is called *Ujjayee*. It can cure dyspepsia, dysentery, fevers, liver and spleen disorders asthma, consumption, chronic bronchitis, etc.

(5) Close the mouth by sitting in the posture known as *Padmasana* and inhale through the left nostril and exhale through the right without holding in the air long. Repeat this ten to sixteen times. This is called *Bhrasrika*. It can cure *thridosha i. e.* ailments caused by Vata (wind), pitta (bile) and (kafa) phlegm. It also improves appetite by curing dyspepsia. (See Ch. IX).

These Breathing exercises stimulate even *Sushumna* nerve, quicken circulation and purify the blood.

Soorya Namaskara or Salutation to the sun.

Some Psychic Exercises with deep breathing to preserve health, and prolong life.

He who wishes to preserve health and prolong life should direct his gaze towards the tip of his own nose, hold the body neck and head straight and without looking to the sides salute the sun 12 times after a bath in cold water thrice a day, morning, noon and evening.

संप्रेक्ष्य नासिकाग्रं च दिशश्चानवलोकयन् ।
समकायशिरोग्रीवो भास्करं प्रणमेत्सदा ॥ ११ ॥

How to salute the Sun.

उरसा, शिरसा, दृष्ट्या, मनसा, वचसा तथा, ।
करद्वयेण, जानुभ्यां, पद्भ्यांच प्रणमेद्रविम् ॥ १३ ॥

Concentrate the mind and the gaze on the sun, then lie postrate on the ground so that the head, chest, both the hands, both the thighs and both the legs touch the ground ; keep breathing deep and utter "O Sun! I salute thee".

"त्रिकालस्नानसंयुक्तः स्वधर्मनिरतस्तथा ।
विध्युक्तकर्मणा नित्यं भास्करं प्रणमाम्यहम्" ॥ १४ ॥

I salute Bhaskar always in the manner prescribed and discharge duties after taking baths thrice a day.

विरक्ताश्च गृहस्थाश्च नत्वा श्रीभास्करं सदा ।
अभूवन् रोगहीनास्ते बलिनः सुखिनस्तथा ॥ १५ ॥

In ancient times both anchorites and married men attained health, strength and happiness by practising salutations to the bright orb of heaven

The sun is said to have 12 aspects, one every time the Earth comes between one of the signs of the zodiac and the *Sun* during its rotation on its own axis. He is thus known to be द्वादशात्मा *The twelve-souled*". He is to be saluted at least 12 times, thrice daily as stated above and after each salutation recite one of the follwing in the order given.

(1) ओं मित्रायनमः Aum Mitraya Namah
(2) ओं रवयेनमः Aum Ravaye Namah
(3) ओं सूर्यायनमः Aum Suryaya Namah
(4) ओं भानवेनमः Aum Bhanave Namah
(5) ओं खगाय नमः Aum Khagaya Namah
(6) ओं पूष्णे नमः Aum Pooshne Namah
(7) ओं हिरण्यगर्भाय नमः Aum Hiranyagarbhaya Namah
(8) ओं मरीचये नमः Aum Mareechaye Namah
(9) ओं आदित्यायनमः Aum Adityaya Namah
(10) ओं सावित्रेनमः Aum Savitre Namah
(11) ओं अर्कायनमः Aum Arkaya Namah
(12) ओं भास्कराय नमः Aum Bhaskaraya Namah

The sound ओं Aum represents sun, water and air.

अकारो द्युतिमानर्क उकार उदकं तथा ।
मकराश्च मरुत्प्रोक्त स्तेषामोङ्कारसम्भवः ॥ १६ ॥

ओं *Aum* is the combination of three letters अ, उ and म· अ A from Arka the sum उ u from udaka the water and ma from मरुत् the Air—These are the three elements or rather the substances in Nature which we need always for the preservation of health and prolongation of life. With this mystic letter *Aum* prefixed to the 12 names of the sum one should salute the Sun thrice daily in the following way at least 12 times on each occasion.

(1) First make a seat 2 feet long and 2 feet broad made up of *Khadi* or any other thick cloth or of a thin

cloth eight-folded. Spread it on soft even ground and then stand erect behind it facing the sun. Make the abdomen tense by inhaling deeply fill out the chest by holding the breath and press the arms against the sides and salute the sun with both the palms touching each other.

(2) Stand erect facing the sun, bend the body without bending the knee-joints and touch the ground with your palms; if you find it difficult, attempt it slowly and touch the ground at least with your fingers and gradually accustom yourself to touch the ground with the palms placed close to the toes, exhale slowly while you bend.

(3) Stand erect facing the sun and stretch your left leg behind; then bend down and touch the ground with your palms without bending your elbow joints and stretch behind the right leg also and then let both the knees touch the ground.

(4) Then prostrate yourself so that your forehead, chest, hands, thighs and legs touch the ground properly. The forehead and the chest may be placed on the afore-said cloth so that they may not touch the ground.

(5) Then stiffen your hands and breathe deeply so that both the lungs and the chest are filled with fresh air as far as possible; then raise the head up, all the weight of the body resting on the hands. Stand up straight by stiffening both the knees. Then salute the Sun as mentioned in the columm (1) above.

These are the five aspects of one salutation. This exercise gives tone to the mind, brains, head, neck, spine, heart, lungs, abdomen, waist and also to arms and legs and preserves health properly.

CHAPTER IX.

EXERCISE

Preventive and Curiative

Exercise is the natural accompaniment of Naturopathy. It favours thermic reaction and imparts energy to the limbs and cheerfulness to the mind. Everything in this universe is in its proper motion and having its due exercisc. Even the sun which we see daily as the largest and brightest luminary in the sky is always moving in its orbit on its own axis. All the planets are moving round it. the Earth we inhabit also is in its motion always like other planets. Trees, plants, creepers, and even the grass are always shaken by the wind. The more they are shaken the stronger they grow and their roots penetrate deeper in the earth. The birds in the air, the beasts on land and the fishes in water are all moving about and having their proper exercise. Human beings also who take proper exercise get stronger and healthier and keep always free from disease.

Nature has so constituted us that regular and proper exercise is neccssary to counteract the wear and tear of life. This wear and tear goes on from hour to hour and day to day and exercise is needed to rebuild the body and re-invigorate the mind every day.

Natural Exercise

(1) Regular open air work in bright sunlight until proper perspiration is induced is the best of all exercises for human beings; digging or tilling the ground for

growing vegetables, fruits, flowers, watering the plants, etc. are the most suitable. Those who have no facilities for such work may take brisk walks in the bright sun till they perspire freely. While walking, the whole body should be erect with shoulders turned backwards; breathing should be vigorous and deep. A healthy young man may need to walk 6 to 12 miles a day; the convalescent, weak persons, and women should at least walk 3 to 5 miles a day.

Physical Exercise

Those who are required to work hard physically are inclined to think that they need no special exercise. This however is a mistake as all physical labour either outdoor such as carrying loads, etc. or indoor such as work in factories, mills, etc. brings only certain parts of the body into action while the other parts remain inactive, and tends to unequal development which is injurious to the body. It is therefore advisible that such persons should take appropriate exercise to develop and strengthen the unexercisied parts of the body. The author does not mean, that they should go through an exhausting course of exercises such as heavy weight lifting, athletic feats, etc. but some mild health preserving exercises, which will promote normal development of all the parts of the body and preserve the health and prolong life.

General Rules for exercise.

(1) When taking any exercise we should face the sun, the God of light, the brightest luminary of heaven so that we may draw some energy from Him.

(2) While taking exercise by lying down we should direct our head to the north towards the Pole Star, the fountain of magnetism so that it may impart some magnetism to us.

(3) We should be bare-headed, barefooted and have as little clothing as possible so that we come in direct touch with mother Earth and her life element fresh air so that we may obtain proper magnetism from her.

(4) Exercise should be taken when the mind and body are at ease and in open places such as gardens, court-yards, verandahs, spacious halls or rooms, near an open window or where there is an uninterrupted current of fresh air.

(5) Do not take any vigorous exercise when you are tired, nor take it until you feel quite tired, nor take it just before or soon after a meal.

(6) Undress yourself or wear a loose light dress so that it does not interfere with the free movements of the limbs and so that all the pores of the body are well-ventilated by the touch of fresh air.

(7) No Apparatus is necessary while taking exercise. But those who feel the necessity may use light wands, clubs, dumb-bells or grip dumb-bells not heavier than one or two pounds.

(8) Begin the exercise each day with a few light movements and gradually try and make it vigorous increasing at the same time the number of movements. If any movements cause pain or uneasiness do them only five times and increase the number gradually.

Caution—Very weak persons and those who suffer from asthma, palpitations, phthisis pulmonalis, tabes mesenterica, hernia, displacement of uterus, fall of rectum or those who are liable to apoplectic fits should not take vigorous exercises except under the supervision of an expert physician.

Head and Neck Exercise.

(1) All proper movements of the head and neck strengthen the vital functions of the whole organism by toning up the muscles of the neck, chest and back. They also cure obstinate headaches, neuralgic pains, obstinate catarrh of the head and chest, dimness of sight, tonsillitis, all sorts of throat troubles, enlargement of cervical glands, etc.

Turning of the head.

(2) Make the neck tense and slowly turn the head toward the left and touch the left shoulder with your chin, then slowly turn the head towards the right side and touch the right shoulder with your chin breathing deep all the while; do it ten to sixteen times.

Rolling of the head.

(3) Place the left hand on the forehead and the right on the occiput and raise the head as high as possible. Then roll the head round as much as possible ten to sixteen times.

Bending the Head Backward and Forward.

(4) stand erect facing the sun, make the neck tense and then slowly bend the head backward and then bend it forward as much as possible. Repeat the process ten

to sixteen times.; breathe deeply during the procedure. Remaining in the same position you can twist the neck and bend the head backward.

Turning and Raising the head.

(5) stand erect facing the sun and raise the head as high as possible making the neck tense as much as possible, and then turn the head to the left slowly then to the right steadily. Repeat this ten to sixteen times breathing deeply all the while. Plate II. Fig. 5.

Sustaining the weight of the body on Head and Neck.

(6) Lie down on a carpet the head and the occiput touching it, the head pointing towards the North Pole and the legs towards the South Pole; make the neck and back tense as much as possible and raise the legs up and stretch them towards the head so that the knees touch the forehead and the whole weight of the body rests on the head and neck; remain in this position as long as possible. Repeat the procedure five to ten times. This is an excellent exercise of the head and neck beneficial to those suffering from dim sight and neuralgic pains.

Chest and Lung Exercise.

(7) Stand erect facing the sun, gently raise the arms, palms pointing upwards and stretch them out firmly as if trying to touch the ceiling; breathe deep 10 to 16 times; inhale while raising the hands and exhale while bringing them slowly down; this will improve the undevloped shoulders, cure the flat or pegion chest, large abdomen, hollow back, etc.

(8) Raise the arms and palms to be in a line with the shoulders and stretch them firmly out-ward and backward; the head thrown somewhat backward and the face pointing towards the ceiling; lift the chest and expand it with deep breath 10 to 16 times. This will broaden and strengthen the chest and shoulders and will cure palpitation of heart.

(9) Keep the arms hanging loosely at the sides and gently inhale, at the same time; raise the arms straight at the sides, when the lungs are full raise the hands so that they meet and the thumbs touch one another and turn the face towards the ceiling. Then without holding the breath exhale gently sweeping the arms and hands down-ward and forward; make these movements slowly and gently; this exercise will cure pain in the chest, sleeplessness, nervousness, headaches, etc.

(10) Raise the hands up to the waist touching the back with the thumbs and bend forward toward the floor; bend 10 to 16 times. Inhale while bending, exhale while rising; do all this gently without effort; this gives strength to the abdomen and the back and cures dyspepsia, flatulence and constipation.

(11) Raise the hands backward touching the back just under the shoulder blades. Then gently incline first the head then the body and bend the chest forward; expand the back and breathe deep 10 to 16 times. Then bend the back towards the chest, not towards the abdomen; breathe deep holding the waist firm and without bending; move the chest and neck thus and breathe deeply 10 to 16 times. This will strengthen the heart

and the chest. This exercise is invaluable for women and those who lead an indoor life. These movements will improve the voice, cure tonsillitis, expand the chest, sterengthen the heart and improve general health. (Pl. II)

To strengthen the muscles of the arms, abdomen, back and waist.

(12) Stand erect facing the sun ; raise both the hands up above the head and bend the body towards the back as much as possible. Then bend forward until the fingers touch the feet, keeping the knees straight. Do it 5 to 10 times twice daily morning and evening. After a few days bend more and more until you are able to touch the ground with your whole palms. Inhale deeply and exhale slowly. See plate II. Fig. 2.

To strengthen the functions of the chest stomach, liver and spleen.

(13) Stand erect facing the sun; raise the right hand up above the head and the left stretching towards the left side only. Then bend to the left as far down as possible. Then assume the original position and raise the left hand up as above as possible keeping the right hand stretched straight towards the right side only and bend the body towards the right side as down as possible. Repeat the process several times. Inhale deeply and exhale slowly.

To strengthen the Chest and increase the Capacity of the Lungs.

(14) Stand erect facing the sun; stretch both the arms backward so that the hands touch each other; try to

bring the hands as high as possible raising them higher with each repetition; rise yourself up standing on the toes and fingers of the feet. Then stretch the arms forward so that the palms touch each other. Inhale deeply while raising the body and exhale slowly while lowering the toes and returning to the original position. Do so 12 to 20 times thrice or at least twice a day.

To strengthen the muscles of the abdomen and to reduce extra fat.

(15) Stand erect facing the sun and keeping the hands on the hips; keep the feet about 6 inches apart. Then bend towards the right side as much as possible and then assume the former position. Then bend towards the left as much as possible and return to the original position. Then bend yourself on the front side as much as possible slowly and steadily and assume the former position. Then bend the back backward slowly as much as possible and resume the original position. Repeat it several times. Inhale deeply and exhale slowly during the exercise. See Plate II. Figure 3.

Exercise for Abdomen and waist.

(16) Lie down on the ground the back touching the earth the head pointing towards the north pole and stretch the legs straight like sticks towards the south pole. Stiffen the abdomen and draw it in as much as possible; slowly raise the head without stretching the hands on the ground and without raising the legs and bend double so that the fore-head touches the knees; if you can't do it touch the soles of both the legs with both the palms bending your waist, but without bending your legs

Then slowly lie down on the earth without resting the hands on the ground; repeat the process ten to sixteen times. This is an exellent exercise for the abdomen and waist. It cures constipation, dyspepsia, flatulence, lumbago, etc.

Exercise for abdomen, waist, and buttocks.

(17) Assume the position mentioned in the Exercise (16), then hold fast with both the hands the lower portions of your thighs so that the palms touch the above portions of the popliteal fossae keeping all the weight of the body on both the hips. Then make slow and steady movements likes a see-saw. This is a good exercise not only for the hands, arms and legs but it is an excellent exercise for strengthening the muscles of the abdomen, waist, hips, etc. It cures dyspepsia, lumbago, pelvic pains, sciatica, rheumatic pains in the knees, etc.

Exercise to Strengthen the Muscles of the shoulders and arms.

(18) Lie down as directed in Exercise No. 16 ; then raise both the hands above the head and bring them flat on the ground; then raise the right hand slowly and steadily and stretch it down; then repeat the procedure with the left hand. Do it at least ten times with each hand; take deep breaths through the nostrils during this procedure; then stretch the hands straight the right hand towards the right side, the left hand towards the left. Then raise the right hand slowly and stretch it over the left; and then take it back to its former position; then raise the left hand in the same way and place it on the right hand flat and then take it back to its former position; do so ten to sixteen times.

This exercise will not only strengthen both the shoulders and the arms but will also cure asthma, cough and palpitations by oxidising the respiratory organs and strengthening the chest.

Exercise to strengthen the legs

(19) Lie down on the ground with the back touching the ground, the head directed towards the North Pole and stretch the legs straight like sticks toward the South Pole. Then slowly and steadily raise the right leg up as high as possible and then bring it down slowly till it touches the ground and do the same with the left leg without bending the knee. Repeat the process ten times or more with both the legs alternately. Then turn to the right side and do the some ten times. Then turn to the left side and repeat the exercise with the left leg ten times. Then lie flat on the ground the abdomen touching the ground and raise the right leg slowly and steadily as much as possible and then bring it down and touch the ground with it. Then raise the left leg in the same way; do it alternately 10 to 16 times.

This exercise will strengthen both the legs and cure epidydimitis and varicocele if other necessary measures are also adopted.

Exercise to Strengthen the Whole Body

(20) Sit down facing the sun, keeping both the feet 15 to 18 inches apart. Do not allow the hips to touch the ground. Then stretch the hands and keep the elbows on the legs just above the knees. Then slowly raise yourself up and stretch down the head as far as the ground, and raise it immediately and stretch

the right knee as far as the ground and then briskly raise it up; stretch the head again down to the ground and raise it immediately and then stretch the left knee down as far as the ground and raise it briskly and stretch the head down as before. Then comes the turn of the right knee and then the head and then the left knee and so on. Repeat this procedure several times. First try 10 to 16 times then gradually increase the number to 100 or 150 or even more if possible. This exercise will cure all diseases and make one strong, hearty and hale. It also prevents all diseases if practised daily twice morning and evening and if possible even at night before going to bed.

PSYCHOLOGICAL EXERCISE

Postures or आसनs as prescribed in the Yoga Philosophy.

आसनैरेव प्राप्नोति । मानवो नाडिशोधनम् ॥
शरीरलाघवं तस्माद् । दृढमारोग्यमेवच ॥ १ ॥

The advantages of yogasanas are:—(1) Cleaning of the body (2)making the body lighter and (3) attainment of perfect health.

नाडिसंशोधनं कुर्या द्युक्तमार्गेण यत्नतः
वृथाक्लेशो भवेत्तस्य तच्छोधनमकुर्वतः ॥ २ ॥

The body, the temple of the human soul, should be made clean, through the proper channels, if it is not cleaned properly a host of ailments will be the result.

शुद्धिमेति यदा सर्वं । नाडिचक्रं मलाकुलम् ॥
तदैव जायते योगी । प्राणसंग्रहणे क्षमः ॥ ३ ॥

When the body and the blood are cleansed of impurities, life will be prolonged by freedom from disease.

युवा वृद्धोऽति वृद्धो वा । व्याधिष्ठो दुर्बलोऽपि वा ॥
अभ्यासात्सिद्धि माप्नेति । प्रोक्तमेतन्मुनीश्वरैः ॥ ४ ॥

The young or the old the sick or the weak will succeed if they persevere. So say the sages.

ब्राह्मणः क्षात्रियो वैश्यः । शूद्रो नारी नरस्तथा ॥
प्राप्नोत्यरोगतां योगात् । शान्ति तेजो बलं धृतिम् ॥ ४ ॥

Brahmin, Kshatriya, Vaishya, or Shoodra, male or female can attain sound health, contentment, brightness, strength and courage from yoga.

मधुरं लघुपाकंच । तथा धातुप्रपोषकम् ॥
मनोभिलाषितं भोज्यं । योगी भोजनमाचरेत् ॥ ५ ॥

A yogi should eat sweet, easily digestible and strength giving food in sufficient quantity.

रुक्षं लवणयुक्तंच । तिक्तमुष्णं तथोत्कटम् ॥
अत्याम्लंच कदन्नंच । नित्यं योगी विवर्ज्ययेत् ॥ ७ ॥

A yogi should always avoid tasteless, salted, bitter, hot and pungent food; also very sour food and bad or unwholesome food stuff.

आसनैः शुद्धिमाप्नोति नारी वा नर एव हि
युवाभवाति वृद्धोऽपि सततं योगसाधनात् ॥ ८ ॥

Both man and woman can cleanse their body with the help of Asanas; by observing the proper methods of yoga; even an old man will attain the energy of youth.

देहे कृशत्वं, नयने च तेजः चित्तेच शान्ति वदनेच कान्तिम्
अरोगताचाग्निप्रदीपनंच योगी सदाविंन्दाति सत्यमेतत्॥ ९ ॥

Translation :—It is true that a Yogi always attains leanness in the body, brightness in the eyes, lustre on the face and calmness in the mind. He also gets his appetite improved and obtains freedom from disease.

आसनानि बहून्येव कथितानि बुधैःपुरा
तेषां लोकहितार्थाय सारमेतद् ब्रवीम्यहम् ॥ १० ॥

Many postures have been prescribed by the learned sages of old; I narrate only the most important ones out of them for the welfare of the people.

(21) नौलिः Nauli a preliminary exercise

आमन्दावर्तयोगेन तुन्दं सव्यापसव्यतः
नतांसो भ्रामयेदेषा नौलिः सिद्धैः प्रचक्ष्यते
मन्दाग्निसन्दीपनकारिणीच तथैव संशोधकरीच नाड्याः
अशेषदोषामयशोषणीच हठक्रिया नौलिरियं निगद्यते

What is called *Nauli* by the siddhas is the successful standing up with bent shoulders keeping the palms on the top of the knees and swinging the abdomen slowly from right to left and left to right a number of times. This *Nauli* prescribed in *Hatha Yoga* is a curer of dyspepsia by stimulating appetite and reliever of constipation. It also cures all the ailments caused by the disorders of humours. (See plate No. III.)

(22) योगासन Yogasana

उत्तानौ चरणौ कृत्वा संस्थाप्य जानुनोपरि
असनोपरि संस्थाप्य उत्तानं करयुग्मकम् ॥ ११ ॥
पूरकै वायुमाकृष्य नासाग्रमवलोकयेत्
योगासनं भवेदेतद्योगिनां योगसाधनम् ॥ १२ ॥

Keep the upper portion of the right foot on the left knee and the upper portion of the left foot on the right knee; and insert the right palm under the right knee and the left palm under the left knee and sit erect in this posture inhale and fill in the lungs with pure air and then exhale slowly and steadily 10 times directing the gaze over the tip of the nose. This position is called Yogasana. At times raise yourself and sustain with your hands.

It purifies the blood, makes the body lighter and overcomes laziness. Plate IV.

(23) सिद्धासन Siddhasana.

योनि स्थानकमंघ्रिमूलघटितं संपीड्य गुल्फेतरम्
मेंढ्रे संप्रणिधाय तं तु चिबुकं कृत्वा हृदिस्थायिनम्
स्थाणुः संयमितेंद्रियोऽचलदृशा पश्यन्भ्रुवोरंतरम्
साधूनांच विधीयते फलकरं सिद्धासनं प्रोच्यते ॥ १५ ॥

Fix the heel of the left feet under the hips and the heel of the right foot below the navel and above the sexual organs; then fix the chin over the upper portion of the chest holding the spine straight and direct the gaze between the two eyebrows. This posture of yoga is called Siddhasana. It keeps the mind calm and quiet, purifies the blood and gives control over passions. This is chiefly recommended for bachelors, widowers and those who are required to observe abstinence on account of the pregnancy, confinement or illness of wife.

(24) पद्मासन Padmasana

वामोरूपरि दक्षिणं हि चरणं संस्थाप्य वामं तथा
दक्षोरूपरि पश्चिमेन विधिना धृत्वा कराभ्यां दृढम्
अंगुष्ठे हृदये निधाय चिबुकं नासाग्रमालोकयेत्
एतद् व्याधिविनाशकारणपरं पद्मासनं प्रोच्यते ॥ १६ ॥

Keep the right foot on the left thigh and the left foot on the right thigh so that both the heels touch close both the groins; then stretch both the hands back and hold fast the right toe by the right hand and the left toe by the left hand; then press the chest with the chin and direct the gaze on the tip of the nose and breathe deeply. This position of Yoga is called Padmasana. It enables one to cure all diseases himself.

(25) भुजंगासन Bhujangasana

अंगुष्ठनाभिपर्यंतमधो भूमौ हि विन्यसेत् ॥
कराभ्यांच धरां धृत्वा । ऊर्ध्वं शीर्षं फणीवहि ॥ १७ ॥
पूरकै रेचकैर्यत्ना । त्प्रणायामंच कारयेत् ॥
भुजंगासन मित्याहु । रेतद्योगविशारदाः ॥ १८ ॥
देहाग्निवर्धकंचैतत् । सर्वरोगविनाशनम् ॥
श्वासकासहरंचैव योगिभिः कथितं पुरा ॥ १९ ॥

Lie down on the ground, the abdomen touching the earth; stretch your hands down as far as your navel then touching the ground with your both the palms raise your head like a cobra; then inhale and exhale on Pooraka and Rechaka methods. This position is called Bhujangasana by expert yogis. It increases the sub-normal temperature to the normal state; it also cures cough, asthma and other respiratory complaints.

(26) मयूरासन Mayurasana

धरामवष्टभ्य करद्वयेन तत्कूर्परस्थापित नाभिपार्श्वः ॥
उच्चासनो दण्डवदुत्थितः स्यान्मयूरमेत त्प्रवदन्ति पीठम् २० ॥
हरति सकलरोगानाशु गुल्मोदरादीन्
अभिभवतिच दोषानासनं तन्मयूरम्
बहुकदशनभुक्तं भस्मकुर्यादशेषम्
जनयति जठराग्निं जारयेत्कालकूटम् ॥ २१ ॥

Lie down on the ground pressing the abdomen to the earth, stretch down both the hands and let both the elbows touch both the sides of the navel. Then touching the ground by both the palms, lift the whole weight, of the body on these two hands which will resemble the two legs of a peacock the whole body should be stretched in a straight line resting on the two hands. This posture is called Mayurasana in Yoga philosophy. It cures several diseases such as enlargement of the liver and spleen and the ailments caused by the vitiation of wata, pitta and kafa (wind, bile and phlegm). It also cures the effects of errors in diet and of bad unnatural food: it also removes auto-toxin generated in the body by objectionable food. Plate V.

(27) वृक्षासन Vrikshasana.

वामोरुमूलदेशेच याम्यं पादं निधायच
तिष्ठेत्तु वृक्षवद्भूमौ वृक्षासनमिदं विदुः ॥ ९२ ॥

Stand up straight on the ground then raise the right foot and touch the left thigh with it as high as possible keeping the balance properly standing on the left leg only. After a while stand on the right leg keeping the balance properly and touching with the left foot the right thigh as high as possible; this posture is called Vrikshasana. This increases the power of balancing and it is very useful for travellers; it also helps to improve digestion and cures asthma.

(28) धनुरासन Dhanurasana

प्रसार्य देहं भुवि दण्डवद् यो । धृत्वा दृढं पादयुगं कराभ्याम्
पृष्ठं धनुस्तुल्यवितर्तितंच करोति यस्मिन् धनुरासनं तत् ।२३।

Lay the body on the ground like a stick, touching it with the abdomen; catch hold of both the legs fast with bc‘h hands right one by the right hand and left one by the left hand bending the back like a bow. This posture is called Dhanurasana. It strengthens the chest, waist, hands and legs. It also improves digestion and cures flatulence and confers briskness and energy.

(29) पश्चिमतानासन Paschimatanasana.

प्रसार्य पादौ भुवि दंडरूपौधृत्वा पदाग्रे सुतरां कराभ्याम्
जानूपरिन्यस्त ललाटदेशोवसेदिदं पश्चिमतानमाहुः ॥ २४ ॥
इति पश्चिमतानमासनाग्र्यं पवनं पश्चिमवाहिनंकरोति
उदयं जठरानलस्य कुर्यादुदरे कार्श्यमरोगतांच पुंसाम् ॥ २५ ॥

Sit down on the ground and stretch both the legs; then hold fast both the toes by both the hands; Then bend down the head so that your forehead touches the knees. This Posture is called Paschimatanasana in Yoga Philosophy. It improves digestion removes flatulence and constipation and reduces the fat surrounding the abdomen thereby reducing the circumference of the abdominal region. It also spreads the wind in Sushumna vein and strengthens it by quickening the circulation and purifying the blood.

योगमुद्रा Yoga Mudra.

(30) महामुद्राविधि: Mahamudravidhi.

पायुमूलं वामगुल्फे संपीड्य दृढयत्नतः
याम्यपादं प्रसार्याऽथ करे धृतपदांगुलिः ॥ २६ ॥
कण्ठसंकोचनं कृत्वा भ्रुवोर्मध्यं विलोकयेत
महामुद्रेति सा प्रोक्ता योगेभिः पूर्वसूरिभिः ॥ २७ ॥
चंद्रांगे तु समासाद्य सूर्यांगे पुनरभ्यसेत्
यावत्तुल्या भवेत्संख्या ततो मुद्रां विसर्जयेत ॥ २८ ॥

क्षयकासमुदावर्तं प्लीहां जीर्णज्वरंतथा
नाशयेत्सर्वरोगांश्च महामुद्राऽतिसेवनात् ॥ २९ ॥

Seat yourself keeping the buttocks over the heel of the left foot; this will require some efforts; stretch the right leg and hold the right toe fast with both the hands. Then stiffen the neck and press the chin over the chest and direct the sight midway between the eyebrows. This position is called Mahamudra by old experienced yogis. This should be done several times in alternation with the right heel being placed under the battocks. Do it the same number of times. This exercise will cure consumption, asthma, liver and spleen troubles, gastric fever, low fever, constipation, flatulence, dyspepsia, etc.

(31) विपरीतकरणीमुद्रा Vipareeta Karaneemudra

शिर्षासन or Shirshasana (Plate Fig.)

करद्वयं शिर आधः ऊर्ध्वं पादद्वयं तथा
करणी विपरीतैषा । चिराभ्यासेन सिध्यते ॥ ३० ॥
अधःशिरश्चोर्ध्वपादः । क्षणं स्यात्प्रथमे दिने
क्षणाश्च किंचिदधिक । मभ्यसेश्च दिने दिने ॥ ३१ ॥
नित्यमभ्यासयुक्तस्य । जढराग्निविवर्धिनी
सर्वरोगहराचेति । योगिभिः कथ्यते पुरा ॥ ३२ ॥
शिरोरोगं नेत्ररोगं । क्षयं कासंच साहरेत्
तस्याःसाधन मात्रेण वृद्धो विन्दाति यौवनम् ॥ ३३ ॥

Translation:—On a soft cushion place the vertex then place both the hands on both sides of the head. Then raise the whole body stretching both the legs straight up sustaining the whole weight of the body on the head and hands and keeping the balance properly. First day do so for a few seconds only and keep increasing the duration daily. This process is said to be useful by old Yogis in improving the appetite and curing dyspepsia; they say that it cures all diseases of the head and eyes and also it makes an old man as energetic as a young man. The author has found it useful in improving the eyesight and curing nervousness. It also cures constipation, urinary and prostatic troubles. It may also restore the original colour to the hair turned prematurely grey.

(32) **विपरीत योगमुद्रा** or **सर्वांगासन.** Vipareeta Yoga-Mudra or Sarwangasana.

Lie flat with the back touching the ground and limbs out-stretched, and the palms touching the sides as low down as possible. Then raise the legs up slowly and steadily the toes pointing upwards, then raise the whole body up, its weight resting on the neck and the head with the hands supporting the waist or with the palms pressing the ground. It is a modified form of *shirshasana* and may be tried by those who cannot practise actual Shirshasana. It has all virtues of Shirshasana and can be tried by any one even children, women and aged persons. It improves digestion, cures nervousness, constipation and dyspepsia, colic, liver and spleen troubles, asthma, cough and weakness of sight. Pl. II. Fig 9.

(33) **विपरीत—अर्धवृक्षासन.** Vipareeta Ardha Vrikshasana.

Assume the above position of Shirshasana and in that position bend your knees and bring down the heels as to touch your hips and remain erect in that position as long as possible. This position is called Vipareeta Ardha Vrikshasana and is as useful as Shirshasana and at the same time it enables one to breathe deep more easily.

CHAPTER X.

Mechano-Therepy or Massage Treatment.

Massage is scientifie rubbing adopted by Naturopaths in the treatment of diseases. It is friction applied systematically to the affected part such as rubbing, stroking, kneading, pressing, pinching, tapping, shaking squeezing, hacking, beating; slapping, etc. to quicken the circulation of blood, to keep the humours in proper condition, to produce warmth and to remove the impurities or useless effete matter from any part of the body. It is employed in inflammatory conditions of any tissue or organ, swellings, abnormal discharges, abnormal growths such as tumours, proud flesh, indurations, granulations, cysts, polypi, papillae, warts, condylomata, emphysomata, etc. It stimulates muscles and glands by producing frictional electricity in them. It not only cures these diseases but also prevents them.

" Static or Kinetic electricity is generated by friction. The process can be best illustrated by an example. When you rub a stick of amber with a piece of silk the amber receives the power of attracting little bits of paper, cork, etc. Resin, glass, sulphur and other things act in the same way " (Platen).

From time immemorial, rubbing of some sort or other has been used by the ancients for curative purposes; our hand naturally and unconsciously rubs the affected part in headaches, injuries and in certain pains. The Chinese have been making use of rubbing for the last 5000 years in healing different diseases.

The Japanese learnt the art from them and brought it to perfection. Hindus have given it a religious garb and have enjoined it on certain days, chiefly on *Diwali* Holiday. In southern India some Ayurvedic physicians try to cure all diseases with massage and bath only.

The Greeks, Romans, Turks, Arabs, Hindoos and Persians are also known to have been making use of massage in paralysis and rheumatism and also to promote circulation. In good old times, the most expert physician as well as the most ignorant barber tried to acquire a knowledge of massage.

"The ancient Greeks and Romans too" says Platen "had a great regard for massage as a valuable method of healing and combined it carefully with hot air baths." Our modern Roman-Irish baths after which the bather was kneaded over the whole body and then rubbed with oil are found to be of great benefit. We find from the scientific treatises of ancient physicians that they fully appreciated the value of the kneading cure. Hippocrates who flourished in the fifth century B. C. studied it thoroughly and was practising it in loosening the stiff joints and in strengthening the relaxed ones. He said that every physician should acquaint himself with the art of "rubbing" for things that have the same name have not always the same effect; rubbing can bind a joint that is too loose and loosen a joint that is too rigid."

Hoffman, physician to the king of Prussia is known to have made use of rubbing in the seventeeth century. In 1813 The Royal Central Institute was established at Stockholm for the use of massage. Dr. Pare in France and Dr. Mezger in Amsterdam deserve all the credit for reviving this method and putting it on a scientific basis; now it has become an essential branch of modern natural and scientific treatment. In America Dr. Mitchell, in 1877, proved its usefulness as an auxilliary treatment in several diseases. William Murrell, von Mosengeil and Dr. Playfair are also known to have practised massage with marvellous results in their days.

Dr. Kellogg of America says that massage may be employed in such a way as to produce sedative as well as tonic and alterative effects of both a remote and a local nature, the same as Hydriatic measures. Rubbing, kneeding, pressing, hacking, tapping with friction and joint movements produce in the body frictional electricity, quicken the circulation, increase the natural warmth, assist the development of the process of tissue change and give tone and strength not only to the nerves but also to the whole body.

The Effects and Advantages of the Massage Treatment.

(1) The circulation of the blood and lymph vessels is promoted.

(2) The blood is drawn up to the upper surface of the skin from the deeper structures; thereby the functional power of the skin is greatly stimulated and improved.

(3) Disorganised matter in the tissues is forced into circulation and easily eliminated from the system.

(4) Assimilation is increased.

(5) Nutrition is improved.

(6) Inflammatory conditions are controlled.

(7) Congestions and thickening of the tissues are reduced.

(8) Pain and stiffness are relieved and a general feeling of well being is noticed.

(9) A dry skin may be moistened and a hot skin may be cooled down with gentle stroking.

(10) Nerves can be stimulated and a feeling of exhilaration produced with a light percussion.

Caution—A deep and forcible massage may produce some abnormal activity of the skin and a percussion with great force and for a longer period than necessary may benumb the nerves and cause exhaustion.

Massage Technique is said to be of passive and active nature; passive movements consist in the straightening or the bending of an arm or leg by manipulating the joints, muscles, blood-vessels, lymphatics and all nerve connections; active movements are done by the patient himself, while the masseur resists or the movements are done by the masseur while the patient puts forth resistence. These active movements act on the muscles and quicken circulation.

In manipulation of the soft tissues of the body, the skin and muscles are rubbed, stroked, kneaded, pounded, pinched, pressed, squeezed, rolled and percussed successively and carefully. The skin underneath which there is a bone must only be massaged with thumbs while the parts which are rich in muscles need stroking.

The Massage is performed in four different ways (always towards the heart, except in lymphangitis of hands, which should be rubbed sideways)—they are denoted as follows:—

(1) Effleurage consists in centripetal stroking or rubbing gently in one direction.

(2) Friction consists in Rubbing with pressure.

(3) Petrissage consists in kneading, wringing, fulling and pinching.

(4) Tapotement consists in tapping, slapping, beating, hacking, clapping, pressing, squeezing, shaking and vibration.

(1) Effleurage.

(1) **Effleurage :**—This movement is done by the tips of the fingers or the palms of hands always towards the heart (except in lymphangitis of the hands) and never away from it. Hence stroke downward from the head to the heart and upward from the arms and limbs. The hand is not lifted at the end of the stroke but glided back to the place where it has started without pressure and without loosing contact with the patient. It quickens the circulation of the blood and lymph vessels.

Stroking Methods of *Effleurage* are performed in the following ways:—

(1) The fingers are held straight and close but not stiffy. The tips or cushions are placed on the part to be worked and a straight upward stroke is made with a little pressure and glided back with no pressure about twenty times. This form is useful in the beginning of

the treatment of neuritis, synovitis of any joint, sprains, strains, etc. Enlarged *glands* and Tubercles also yield to this procedure.

(2) The whole palmar surface may be utilised and the movements performed in the same way when pain is a bit less and in oedema of the legs.

(3) The thumb is separated from the fingers and placed across the top of the hand with fingers underneath the limb being, as it were, held in the hand the movements are done as before. This method is more useful for the limbs of young children.

(4) The Masseur should use both of his hands by placing one on each side of the affected limb of his patient and perform circular stroking movements slowly and steadily with moderate speed and strength on both sides. Dislocation of shoulders, knees, etc. yield wonderfully to these forms of movements. They reduce fat also in obesity.

Note—During the process of massage the patient should practise deep-breathing to stimulate the internal blood and lymph vessels as it helps a good deal to oxidise the blood and hasten the cure of any ailment. The masseur should always begin his massage seance with Effleurage in all acute cases to hasten circulation and diminish inflammatory condition.

(2) Friction or Rubbing.

Friction or **Rubbing** is undertaken by palms or by fingers only of one or both hands as the case may require.

The method of practising Friction.

Movements are made with the cushion of the thumb, the tips of the fingers or with the palms of the hands by placing them over the skin or tender joint with rotatary motion. After ten circular movements have been made, the thumb, finger or hand is moved upward to the next place but without dragging the skin. This process is most effective in squeezing out the products of inflammation and in facilitating absorption and stimulating local circulation. Friction is always followed by Effleurage.

Friction should be carefully learnt and practised by Masseurs to get the best effects in toning up the muscles of the face, neck and bust. It can produce disintigration of tissues and break them up and turn them up 'in small particles and promote re-absorption very effectively. It also spreads the inflammatory products over a larger surrounding area so that they are more readily removed in the blood-stream.

The masseur should clearly understand that the more recent the inflammatory condition with more the serous substances the more effective is the effleurage; and the older the inflammatory products are with more the fibrinous and cellular elements, the more does the friction show its value in producinlg the beneficial effects.

Caution—Friction is contra-indicated in the neighbourhood of all purulent processes and in all pus-formations.

The frictions are of three sorts:—

(1) In *centripetal* friction the movements are made in the direction of the blood current in the veins, say-for instance, for legs from below upwards (except in the coldness of extremeties) and for hand towards the body; fingers or palms may be utilised for the purpose.

(2) In *Centrifugal* friction movements are made opposite to that of the blood current.

(3) In *Circular* friction circular movements are made to increase warmth for instances on the head, shoulders, buttocks, joints, knees, palms, feet, etc.

Procedure to be Adopted in Friction.

1. Head—from above down-wards
2. Neck—downward.
3. Shoulderblades—circular
4. Back—down and circular
5. Hïps—circular
6. Chest—sternum to axilla
7. Abdomen upper—downward
8. Abdomen lower—downward and sideways.
9. Arms and legs—from below upward.
10. Palms and soles—circular

Special Hints for Friction.

(*a*) In rheumatism and neuralgia the friction should not be vigorous.

(*b*) In paralysis, faulty circulation and itching skin the friction should be vigorous.

(*c*) In eruptive fever friction should be avoided.

(*d*) After a hot, warm or neutral bath, friction is not necessary.

(*e*) If the patients cannot bear cold water, oil may be used or friction on the dry skin may be tried.

By its power of causing re-absorption of inflammatory products, massage, especially Friction helps to loosen or stretch parts which have become stiff or shortened on account of inflammatory condition or those which have become adherent to other parts such as scar contractions, peritoneal adhesions between the bowels, fixation of the uterus by parametric or perimetric exudation.

Friction is of great therapeutic value in connection with haematoma, cellulitis of muscles, tendons, joints, capsules, ligaments and fascia, and also in the nerve trunks in the case of interstitial neuritis.

Just as a piece of iron or steel is magnetised when rubbed by a magnet, so the patient gets the latent electro magnetic energy or the vital power roused up in his body by massage. The patient forms a negative pole while masseur forms a positive one during the course of massage; stronger the masseur physically, mentally and morally the better results will be produced in the patient.

Friction for Preserving Health.

For those who cannot take proper exercise and for those who cannot take early morning cold water friction bath, rubbing the whole body with oil is an efficient means of preserving health. Every persons in sound health may try it at least once a week. The ancient Hindoos were in the habit of rubbing their whole body with cocoanut or sesame oil for an hour or so and then taking a hot water bath, which they called (अभ्यंगस्नान) *Abhyanga Snâna* ". Even in these days of western civilization every Hindoo takes such a bath at least once a year during the Divali Festival. The old Romans always had their body rubbed with oil after a bath. The natives of less civilized parts of Africa are still in the habit of rubbing themselves with oil. After a tepid or warm bath the best effects are produced by rubbing the body with oil as the epidermis then absorbs it readily; care should however be taken not to apply too much oil. When the body is massaged the oil will be properly absorbed by the skin; the surplus oil may be removed by finally rubbing the body with a soft towel. cocoanut oil and sesame oil are the best. Some allopathic doctors are of opinion that Codliver oil is the best for consumptive patients and rickety children as it contains some iodine; but its too strong foul smell may prove it forbidding. The author finds fresh cocoanut juice the best of all things in any case. In emaciation and consumption and rickets it is an excellent application for the skin. Even healthy persons will find it delightful.

Electric Friction Bath

Electrified water may be prepared by exposing a tumbler full of water to the heat of the sun for two or three hours during midday. This water may be rubbed over the painful parts. It is useful in earache, toothache, stiffneck, back-ache, lumbago, rheumatism, etc., and may be of great service for gargling in scurvy, or pyorrhoea, and as a compress over boils, abscesses, carbuncles, painful and indolent ulcers, injuries, sores, burns, scalds, etc, etc; a four-fold linen dipped in the electrified water and placed over the effected part is called a compress. It is an excellent remedy for palpitation, angina pectoris, hepatitis, splenitis, metritis, nephritis, etc. Those who are of subnormal temperature will do well by bathing in Electrified water prepared in a large tub or an Earthen or metal pot by exposing it to the sun as mentioned above.

Acidulated Friction Bath

In Europe and America hydrochloric or sulphuric acid is used to acidulate water. There are also some natural acid springs in America. The author recommends the juice of fresh lemons to be added to water. The patient should sit in the tub and apply friction to his body especially to the lower part of his abdomen. These baths remove constipation and flatulence and are good for congestion of liver or any part of the body. They are also useful for the disorders of the urinary organs. They improve the activity of the skin and are useful for many skin complaints, such as scabies, eczema, pruritus, etc.

The dry Pack with Friction.

In dry packing the patient is wrapped in a large thick woollen blanket in such a way that no air should pass inside and touch his body. A cold compress is applied to the head so that the blood may not rush towards it and a large covering is placed over the covered blanket before the windows are opened and the patient is to be given a wine-glassful of pure cold water every ten or fifteen minutes.

Dry packing is useful in catarrh, influenza, rheumatism, gout and in some chronic diseases where the patient does not perspire. After the patient got sufficient perspiration he should be bathed or his body sponged in tepid water (86 to 90) and then he should be asked to take open air exercise or his whole body must be rubbed over to quicken circulation.

Caution:—Weak and anaemic patients should avoid the dry pack.

It is recommended in Ayurvedic Medical system for catarrhal fever.

शैत्ययोगेन संतापो । विनिर्याति शरीरतः ॥
उष्णवस्त्रादियोगेन । तद्गतिः प्रतिरुध्यते ॥

(3) Petrissage.

Petrissage consists in Kneading, Rolling, Pinching and Fulling. Its physiological effects resemble those of **Friction** in that it promotes absorption of the products of inflammation and those of Tapôtement in that it acts as a muscle stimulus.

In Petrissage or deep massage (1) the muscles and other tissues are stretched and lifted from the bone. (2) The nerves, blood-vessels, lymph vessels, glands and all tissues are stimulated in their function. (3) By the alternate compression and expansion brought about by pressure, lymph is forced out of the spaces and into the lymphatic ducts ; (4) veins are also filled and emptied alternately so that impure blood is sent outward and a supply of fresh blood favoured. To accomplish all this, manipulation must be deep. The muscles must be thoroughly gripped and well-kneaded. This does not mean that force should be used ; it is never necessary.

The Methods of performing Petrissage.

(1) **Kneeding :** With one thumb and index finger any single muscle or muscles are grasped ; the finger is kept steady and muscle is rolled back on it with the thumb. This is done five to ten times, then a very slight onward movement is made and the kneading is repeated.

(2) **Deep kneeding** is performed just as above ; but all the fingers are utilised. The muscles are grasped firmly between the fingers and the ball of the thumb and then squeezed, rolled and kneeded thoroughly and systematically so that every portion of the limb receives its share of this stimulating massage.

(3) **Wringing** :—Hold the limb in two hands one in advance of the other; the hands are twisted backwards and forwards carrying the muscles with them; the movement is very much as a wet cloth is being wrung, it is very useful for the limbs of children suffering from infantile paralysis, and for those who suffer from acid conditions.

(4) **Fulling :**—One hand is placed under a limb, palm upwards; the other over it, palm downwards, and exactly above the first hand. Then a rapid to and fro movement is made on the affected limb with both hands, as one does in warming the hands by rubbing the palms against each other. This method is very useful in over-

coming stiffness and a tendency of getting cramps in the calves or stiffness in the arms and wrists. It is also useful for old people whose circulation is faulty.

(5) **Pinching**—Every one knows how to pinch; but the scientific pinching of the skin and tissues immediately beneath the skin is the most suited for the cure of obesity. It can be tried by stout persons themselves. In squeezing the fat out of the tissues the structures are taken up between fingers and thumbs which should work alternately in a rolling motion. At the same time the tissues should be pressed and squeezed. This form of systematic pinching should be tried twice or thrice a day at least for half an hour each time. It is not only useful for obesity but also for goitre, cyst, fatty tumour, etc. if followed by sunbath.

Caution—Petrissage is very useful for relieving the pains of stiffneck, lumbago, rheumatism, sciatica, etc. But it should not be carried to excess, as it will do more harm than good.

(4) Tapotement of Tapping

Tapotement or Tapping is performed either with the tips of fingers, the palmar surface of the fingers, the hollow of the palms or the sides of the hands. The thumbs should be held upwards and far away from the surface being treated. The movements should be of light springy touch; the hands should be swinging from the wrist and should not be raised more than an inch from the patient's body. Shoulders, abdomen, thighs, buttocks or back may be vigorously tapped and a capillary circulation may be stimulated in those parts and sluggish nerves may be brought to increased action.

The movements being characterised by their blow-like nature are termed as Slapping, Beating, Hacking, Clapping, Vibration and Shaking. They stimulate muscles, nerves and protoplasm of all cells especially of gland cells.

The Methods of performing Tapotement.

(1) **Slapping**:—The palmar surface of the fingers is held straight and close together and the affected muscle is struck transversely, evenly and rhythmically, moving backward and forward in all directions, leaving no parts untouched.

(2) **Beating** is done with the ulnar side of the closed hand (fist).

(3) **Hacking** or chopping—The ulnar border of the open hands and fingers are used. The hands are held a little apart, the palm towards palm, the fingures separated and held loosely fall together at each blow ; the hands strike alternately.

(4) Clapping is done with the whole palmar surface of the hands striking alternately ; the palms are contracted so as to form a hollow or a cup.

(5) **Pressing**—Every one is familiar with pressing. Whenever one receives an injury one's hand naturally goes to the injured part for the purpose of pressing it. It can be done with the palm of the right hand and then leaving the part suddenly and then repeating the process as required.

(6) **Squeezing** is done by holding the part with all the fingers and by pressing it with the thumb rapidly backwards and forwards.

15

(7) **Shaking** is done on the body or a part of the body. In the latter case a hand or foot in an extended position is taken and the whole limb shaken. In the former, the hand is placed on the abdomen and shaken with firm pressure.

(8) **Vibration** is the only manipulation where an instrument called *Vibrator* may be utilized. The manipulation can be performed by fingers as well. The ends of the fingers or the knuckles of the closed hands or the palmar surface of the hands are placed on some parts of the patient's body. A trembling sensation is conveyed to the part through the hand of the masseur.

Note :—Tapping should be followed by a short vibration or shaking. If liver, stomach or abdomen is being treated the vibration should be vigorous, the entire palm of the hand should be used as a base. In rheumatic troubles of the joint, arms and legs must be straightened and doubled several times if necessary.

Caution :—Masseur should be very careful in performing tapping in rheumatism, synovitis, sciatica, stiff-neck, etc. not to make any such movements as would cause pain to the patients. Slow movements with sunbaths have produced marvellous results under the instructions of the author.

Massage may be either general or local. In general massage the masseur manipulates the whole body except the head; he begins with the foot with strokings with one hand or kneading with his thumbs; then he proceeds with the legs, then the arms, then the chest, then the abdomen and lastly the back. Masseur should begin on the first day with left foot and leg and finish off within 20 to 25 minutes gradually increasing the time to an hour.

In local massage a single part of the body is treated at a time according to the need of the patients.

Massage of the head.

(1) Make the patient sit firmly and comfortably

(2) Hold his forehead with the left hand and stroke the head with the right hand the back part cf the head first and then the top or vertex

(3) Friction with one hand, supporting the head with the other hand slowly and steadily

(4) Try hacking with both hands making circles first on the top of the head then on the back of the head and sides.

Head ache, neuralgic pain and depression of mind can be cured by these methods.

Massage of the neck and throat.

(2) The patient should stand or sit facing the masseur with the head thrown back so as to expand his neck. The masseur places his hands at the lobes of the ears and strokes downward to the shoulder; during the massage the patient should breathe deeply and freely. This operation will increase circulation in the veins of the neck and cure stiffneck and other troubles of the neck and also enlargement of the thyroid gland. The author had an occasion to treat and watch a case of goitre with Homeopathic medicines and masssage. The patient was over 40 years of age with a lot of grey hair. It was a surprise to her and her relatives to find that her

grey hair turned black after the cure without the use of any hair preparations. It shows that the thyroid gland has much to do with the colouring matter of the hair.

Massage of the arm

(1) The patient may lie or sit down

(2) Stroke with one hand from wrist to ankle holding fast the wrist with the other hand

(3) Then stroke from the wrist to the shoulder joint.

(4) Friction with the thumb on the extensors and fingers.

(5) Friction with the thumb, the flexors and the fingers.

(6) Knead with both the thumbs upon different muscles chiefly upto extensors and flexors and also biceps and triceps

(7) Hack over the whole arm.

(8) Repeat the process over the other arm also in the same way,

Massage of the Chest

(1) Lay the patient flat on the back placing the arms at the sides.

(2) Stroke with both the hands placing the palms on the sternum. Stroke upward and downward with circular movements.

(3) Stroke with your thumbs over pectorales from sternum towards arms.

(4) Knead with the thumb and fingers steadily if the muscles are paralysed.

(5) Hack around the heart very carefully in case of weakness, dilatation, palpitations of the heart, etc.

(6) Always make the patient breathe deep through nostrils and never through mouth.

Massage of the female breast

Always massage the breast by keeping the hands towards the nipple.

Always use frictions with the tips of the fingers whenever there is hardness in the breasts or whenever they are distended.

Always finish the process with "fulling" with a very gentle pressure with both hands from the base of the breasts upward towards the nipple.

In cracked nipples and coldness of the breast use cocoanut juice mixed with camphor spirits. In undeveloped breasts and dwindled breasts use cocoanut juice with tincture Sabal serrulata and in tumours use cocoanut juice with tincture Phytolacca.

Massage over the liver

(1) The patient should lie on his left side and masseur should sit at his right side

(2) Friction in circles with the palm of the right hand the whole rigion of the liver

(3) Knead the same part with the heel of the hand.

(4) Friction over the different lobes gently and carefully

(5) Make the patient breathe deeply.

(6) In all liver disorders the patient should avoid all oily and fatty substances and fried preparations and should take easily digestible food, milk, fruits, etc.

Massage over the spleen

(1) The patient should be on his right side

(2) The performance is similar to that of liver treatment

Massage of the abdomen

(1) The patient should evacuate his bladder and bowels and then lie flat on his back without any pillow, with his knees drawn up.

(2) Friction from right to left over the region of navel in circle several times gently, gradually increasing the strength.

(3) Kneed over the whole abdomen with the heel of the right hand avoiding all sore and painful places. All hard lumps of faecal matter should be gently broken up with the tip of the fingers, chiefly near the sigmoid flexure; make the patient breathe deeply while massaging his abdomen.

(4) The part below navel should be rubbed very carefully for a long time in all abdominal troubles, such as pain, flatulence, constipation, etc.

Massage of the back.

(1) The patient should lie on his abdomen touching the ground, keeping his arms at the sides.

(2) Stroke with both the hands, one on each side of the spine from the head towards the sacrum.

(3) Friction with the hand one side at a timc.

(4) Knead with both the thumbs keeping one on each side of the spine and friction gently all the spinal nerves

(5) Hacking, pinching, clapping, etc. may be tried according to the needs and discretion of the masseur.

(6) Stroke in the end again very gently, if the patient is weak and if soothing effect is desired; stroke quickly if stimulation is desired.

Massage of the Glutei

(1) The patient should stand bending his body forward holding with his hands a chair or a table or he may lie down flat with his abdomen touching the bed.

(2) Stroke with both the hands, the whole back and spine from the neck downward to the lumbar region

(3) Friction with the hand both the sides

(4) Beat in circles both the sides.

Massage of the prostate gland

After evacuating the bowels and the bladder the patient should lie on his back holding himself his sexual organs stretched up towards his abdomen. Stroking with friction is carefully practised on the perineum by the masseur. The author had tried this method on a young student who had the habit of masturbation and whose hair had grown grey prematurely. After the cure, his hair turned black without any application of dyes or hair oils. This shows that the prostate supplies nutrition to the hair roots through the blood.

In Europe and America some masseurs insert their index or mid-finger in the anus of the patient and hold the prostate fast and perform stroking and frictions with the thumb and fingers of the other hand. The author has never tried this method as yet and does not recommend it as there are some Homeopathic medicines which yield more satisfactory results when administered through the mouth. After the above mentioned cure by chance the author got half a dozen patients with enlarged prostate but two of them had fistula and four of them had venereal disease; so, the author tried homeopathic drugs on them instead of massage treatment. As the result was marvellous, *i. e.* more satisfactory than massage treatment, the author undertakes to cure patients suffering from enlarged prostate with Homeopathic medicines only. See chapter XII.

Massage of the leg

(1) The patient should be made to recline on a sofa or a bed and the masseur should sit towards his sides.

(2) Stroke the foot, sole and dorsum with the palm of one hand grasping the ankle with the other hand.

(3) Stroke with both hands from ankle to hip.

(4) Friction with the thumb on the outer part of the leg from ankle to knee joint.

(5) Then friction with the thumb the inner and outer side of the thigh thoroughly so that all the different muscles are properly acted upon.

(6) Knead with both the thumbs upon the different muscles of the leg.

(7) Hack over the whole leg avoiding the bory portion.

(8) Then perform the same operation on the other leg also.

Rheumatism, paralysis, dropsical swellings, sprains, strains, etc. require the above methods.

Massage is contra-indicated

in (1) wounds (2) burns (3) erysipelas (4) acne (5) eczema (6) malignant tumours (7) suppurations and (8) acute bone diseases.

It is also contra-indicated during

(1) menstruation (2) during pregnancy, (3) during any haemorrhages and in the (4) advanced cases of lymphangitis.

The masseur should not use too much pressure so as to cause discomfort to the patient; massage always be performed on the nude skin.

The masseur's hand should be lubricated with cocoanut juice or oil; olive oil, sweet almond oil or sesamum oil may also be used, but very moderately.

After the massage the massaged part may be exposed to the strong sun for a few minutes or may be covered well for some time.

CHAPTER XI.

Natural and Rational living.

To be healthy we should no longer seek doctor's advice but study Nature and be guided by our own instinct and our organs of sense.

(1) Healthy Residential Places.

The most suitable and healthy place for the residence of human beings is neither a busy and bustling town nor a gloomy and horrid forest; neither a roaring and noisy seashore nor a calm and serene riverside; neither a deep and shady valley nor a whistling and chirping green field. Such places do not seem to be suitable for them. The high and charming peaks and slopes of mountains only seem to be suitable for them. According to the Hindu Mythology our primitive man *Manu* (not the lawgiver of the Hindus but the first known created human being after whom all the human beings are called *Manavas*) with his beloved *Dhavâ* (wife) lived happily in a garden called "*Udyan*" on a peak of a mountain which is still called "*Adam's peak*" as he was called so later on by Brahma the creater.

I quote this story here, neither to refute the Evolution theory of Darwin nor to refute statements of any religious writers of other Faiths who seem to have borrowed this story and introduced it in their religious books with a lot of changes in it, but to prove that the peaks and slopes of mounts are only suitable for the residence of human beings. The story is very old and it is from one of the old Hindu Puranas. It runs thus:—

The first human being was created by Brahma the creator, and was made to live in an " Udyan " (Garden) on the peak of a mount in an island called *Lanka* or *Sinhala Dweep*, the present Ceylon where that mount still exists and its peak is still called " *Adam's peak*"

He was made to live in that garden which contained trees, creepers and plants bearing different kinds of flowers, fruits and nuts in different seasons. He was endowed with one *Dhavà* (wife), *Dhànya* (grains) and *Dhenû* (cow). That garden contained neither a palace nor a hut. He had to live under the shade of trees only which yielded him sweet fruits. The ground was not required to be tilled; still *Dhànya* grew abundantly which was later on called *Neewar* which is now-a-days called " *Rajgira* "

Though the garden was fertile and looked splendid with fresh air, pure water and bright sunlight he had no clothes, no shoes and no furniture; so he had to remain naked,walk bare-footed and sit and lie down on the ground only.

Being tired of this monotonous life they thought of seeing other lands and travelled to the north where they found a large supply of salt water ebbing and falling according to the movements of the moon. He piled up large stones and built a bridge and both of them crossed that bridge which is still called " *Adam's Bridge* " and came to a larger country (now called Hindusthan). Brahma came to know of this and stood before him and exclaimed. " Thou *Adam* ! अदम ! (Sanskrit for the impatient the one having no patience, दम means patience in Sanskrit) you have both disobeyed me and I shall punish you both for your disobedience. Dhava at once prostrated before Brahma and said "My Lord ! Do punish me because I started the idea of seeing far-off lands and I was the cause of all this; but do not punish my loving innocent mate." Manu prostrated before Him and said "My Lord ! Pray punish me but not my tender partner who is too weak to bear the pain of your punishment. It was I who piled up big stones in that expanse of water and built that bridge and helped her to come here, she would not have been able to do all this; therefore forgive her and punish me "

The good old Brahma said—"My good Adam Manu (Impatient Manu) I am pleased with your mutual love soliciting punishment for your own self and requesting me to forgive the other. I forgive you both. Go-on, travel and occupy the whole world. Breathe well, eat well and multiply well. I blame you only for your impatience. I created the whole world for you and for your progeny only, but I wanted you to live in that Udyan on the peak of that mount which is the best and a healthy place to live in."

Since then this Manu was known as Adam Manu, *i.e.,* impatient Manu to distinguish him from other *Manus,* as there were several other Manus also-स्वयंभूमनु (*Swayambhu Manu*). Self-born Manu. वैवस्वतमनु (*Waiwaswat Manu*). Sun-born Manu. Law giver Manu, etc.

According to the usage in sanskrit *Adam's* descendants are all known as *Adami's* आदमि; the word Dhava was corrupted into *Hava*, Ava, Eva and Eve. In southern India the word Ava is still used while addressing a mother and all Hindustani speaking people use the word *Adami* for man, while Marathee and canarese speaking persons use the word *Manava* or *Manushya* for man.

चित्तस्य निग्रहः सम्यग् दम इत्येव कथ्यते ।
दमहीनोऽदमश्चेति विद्वद्भिरभिधीयते ॥

दम-control of mind, *i.e.*, curbing it from temptations and evil propensities ; अदम is one who cannot control them.

This shows that the best residential place for human beings is a garden on the peaks or slopes of mountains much above the sea level. The ancient Aryans too lived on the mountain called Hindukush in Persia.

Those persons styled as Demigods, Yakshas, Gandharvas and Kinnaras all lived on the Himalayas ; Bhils, Kirats and other strong mountain races lived on Vindhya, Meru, Mandara, Malaya and Dardura mountains; they were in those days very strong and healthy beings free from disease.

There they got an ample supply of ozone and pure air which kept their blood pure. Thus they were free from all diseases and disease germs.

This shows that human beings should spend as much of their time as possible in gardens under the shade of trees inhaling fresh air charged with the sweet fragrance of flowers and not in ill-ventilated schools, factories, lecture-halls, billiard rooms, mills, theatres, cinema buildings, opera-houses, etc, where the air is charged with effluvia and nicotine fumes.

(2) Natural and Healthy Sleeping places.

In hot seasons the best place to lie down in and sleep in during the night is under the bespangled canopy of heaven in the craddle of the earth on sandy beds or beds made of soft clean earth on which some clean clothes are spread. Houses are suitable in rainy and snowy days if well-ventilated and not otherwise. While sleeping, one should place one's head towards the north Pole star and one's feet towards south. This position will cure melancholia, sleeplessness, headaches, neuralgic pains in the head, nervousness, etc, The Pole star is the greatest fountain of Electricity, Magnetism, etc.

(3) Natural and Health Preserving Dress.

Premitive man knew no clothes. The earliest cover he sought for his body was of large leaves and later on "*Valkalas*" or clothes made from the bark of certain trees which kept his body exposed to fresh air and bright sunlight. He washed his skin with fresh cold water. These natural habits kept him strong and hale and free from disease. Multiplicity of dress is the product of western civilization and interferes with healthy functions of the skin. As the pores of the body also inhale oxygen from the air the dress worn should be such as will not impede free movement and will help to ventilate freely the pores and oxidise the blood and afford great relief to the lungs.

(4) Natural Method of cleaning the body.

The body must be kept perfectly clean by bathing it daily in cold water as supplied by Nature morning and evening and rubbing it all the while thoroughly and briskly. The practice of applying scented oils to the hair and bathing by pouring hot water on the shoulders and of making use of scented soaps which is prevalent among the refined ladies in India is from hygienic and sanitary points of view most objectionable.* The whole body including the head must be washed thoroughly every day. If the colon, skin and head be kept clean the human hair will impart a pleasant odour and there will be no need for artificial essences of scents. But if these are not kept clean even the scented oil will soon begin to stink when applied to the unclean hair and unhealthy hair-roots; further essences of scents are injurious to the skin and hair roots and they cause certain skin diseases; under their use the hair either begins to fall off or to get prematurely grey. Fresh flowers worn in clean hair will impart the most pleasant odour to the hair which will in every way be pleasing without causing any injury to the skin or hair roots. If a little oil be felt necessary pure and fresh cocoanut,

---

*"Today we use soap made of the fat of animals that have perished from all sorts of diseases ; that is the filthiest material concievable to cleanse our skin. But strictly speaking the skin is not cleansed by the use of soap but rather defiled. The corrosive substances contained in soap always injure the skin. If men were to discard the use of soap in their daily ablutions they would be much cleaner. Those who wash themselves with pure, clean water will be as clean as they need to be. Besides sand is a natural cleaning material." (A Just). Soap-nuts are natural and best.

seasame, almond or olive oil may be applied and the hair washed clean next day with a little lather produced from the soapnuts which are far superior to all scented soaps.

A judge's wife was suffering from an obstinate skin disease; she had tried the best doctors' prescriptions, the best ointments and the best scented soaps; but the skin disease never yielded. A Homeopathic remedy internally and the use of soapnuts externally as adviced by the author cured the skin disease radically; since then she has stuck to soap nuts only. She was known to frequently remark that the natural soap though without any fragrance is far better than artificial scented soaps.

(5) Natural wholesome Food.

Fruits, berries, nuts, milk and cereals are excellent natural food stuffs. Primitive races subsisted on these and never suffered from constipation or diarrhoea. They ate no salt no sugar nor any boiled or fried foods; they ate no spiced preparations nor drank any tea, coffee, soda, syrup, wine or liquors and hence never suffered from any disease; more than ninety percent of the diseases from which civilized nations now suffer are due to errors in diet; excesses, all the artificially preserved food stuffs and highly spiced dishes now supplied on the tables by expert cooks are also the cause of disease.

Of all fruits, the plantain is the best and most wholesome natural food that Nature produces for human consumption. Hindus consider it as the fruit worthy of being offered to God. Old Jews called it *musa paradisica i. e.* the fruit of paradise. Its peculiarity is that it contains no seed to propagate its species. New plantain trees emerge from the bottom of the old plantain trees. The fruit is within the reach of the human hand ; it breeds no worms even if it gets rotten ; it is available in all the seasons ; hence it is plain that it is meant by Nature for human consumption only. Besides it contains natural sugar and all the nutritious salts and vitamins required for the building up of the human body; mangoes, jack-fruits, apples, custard-apples, oranges, sweet limes, peaches, caryca papayas, apricots, dates, figs, grapes, pears, chikoos, jambs, plums, prunes, lakuchees, lachees, Kharbuj's, pine-apples, water-melons, and other fruits are excellent food-stuffs if consumed in their proper season.

So also ordinary berries, craneberries, gooseberries, buckleberries, jambuls, mulberries, raspberries, strawberries, and other sorts of berries are very wholesome if partaken in their proper season.

Among the nuts almonds, charolees, cocoanuts, *beheda* nuts, chest nuts, horse chest nuts, hazel-nuts, kola-nuts, ground-nuts, kajunuts, pistachio and walnuts are the most sustaining and bone forming food-stuffs supplied by Nature for human consumption. They can be used in any season dried in the sun and preserved. They supply a normal quantity of fat to the body and help to keep up the normal and natural heat.

Of all the nuts the cocoanut is the most excellent foodstuff Nature offers to human beings. It contains sweet water rich with nutritive salts and a natural supply of sugar. The nut itself contains white juice resembling milk, which is a better food than the milk of cattle being more nutritive than all other foods. It is better than curds, ghee, codliver oil, eggs and many other nutritive substances recommended by doctors for weak persons and consumptive patients. One large Cocoanut can sustain a man for full 24 hours. Its juice has a better taste than milk itself. It can be safey recommended to every sick person who can not digest milk, as well as to those who have a dislike for milk. It has saved the life of many consumptive patients and rickety children in the experience of the author.

Sugarcane is another food adjunct very useful and very nutritious. It not only quenches thirst but also serves to digest food and to cure flatulence. It is recommended to those suffering from dyspepsia, flatulence and constipation and to all patients in their convalescence from any debilitating disease.

Pomegranets also quench thirst and are most suitable for patients suffering from diarrhoea, dysentery and sprue.

•Sour lemon is another gift of Nature which serves as a remedy to quench thirst and also to cure the worst type of acidity, sour belching, rheumatism, gout, etc.

Spinach, cabbages, cauliflower and other vegetables contain a large quantity of inorganic salts which can be termed as positive mineral elements while they contain very little starch, sugar, protein and other organic substances. Hence they can be termed as positive food materials.

Wheat and other cereals contain a large quantity of starch, sugar, fat, protein and other organic substances and less of positive mineral substances, or what are termed as inorganic substances; hence they can be termed as negatave food substances.

All fruits are rich in both sugar and inorganic salts, hence they can be termed as neutral food substances and are always wholesome and beneficial.

(1) *Acid fruits* such as grapes, oranges, under ripe sweet limes, sour limes, mangoes, apples, pine-apples, sour apples, pomegranates, etc. are ideal eliminators and excellent blood purifiers. An exclusive acid fruit diet for 3 or 4 weeks will surely succeed in eliminating the most irritating poisons from the body and render the patient healthy and free from any disease. Dyspepsia, flatulence, flatulent colic, liver troubles, pustular skin eruptions, obesity, rheumatism, gout, septic poisoning, intestinal toxemia, chronic nasal and intestinal catarrh, etc. have yielded wonderfully to an exclusive diet of these fruits.

(2) *Sweet fruits* such as plantains, custard-apples (Seetafal, Ramafal, etc.) sweet apples, *lachees*, pears, jack-fruits, sweet prunes, sweet limes, dates, figs, melons, mangoes, etc. are less potent as eliminators of poisons from the blood but are more refreshing and more strength-giving than acid fruits; they contain more starch and more albuminous substances and are to be used to build up and strengthen the body.

(3) *Leafy* vegetables such as spinach, lettuce, celery, beet tops, asparagus, cabbages, cauli-flower, radish leaves, etc. are richer in tissue salts which are highly organised in them than the fruits above-mentioned. They are useful to preserve alkaline substances in the blood. They should be eaten fresh and raw in small quantities without salt and spices. If the taste is not liked, grated cocoanut, onion pieces and sour lime juice or a little honey may be added to them.

(4) Under ground vegetables such as roots, potatoes, sweet potatoes, tubers, radishes, ground nuts, etc. should be eaten raw; they may be grated and eaten with grated cocoanut, pieces of onions and sour lime juice. They abound in tissue salts and vitamines and serve as intestinal cleansers and blood purifiers. They also eliminate uric acid from the blood.

(5) Nuts such as walnuts, kajunuts (Anacardium occidentalis), pistachio, almonds, charolees, cocoanuts chest nuts, etc,, are rich in oily or fatty substances; they are very difficult to digest unless well masticated and properly insalivated, they are very useful foodstuffs for those who are weak, lean and of subnormal temperature; they help to keep up the original body heat and also to increase it up to the normal. They should be eaten raw without sugar or salt, after being soaked in fresh water for some hours.

Note :—Garlic and onion are considered as *Tamasi* food by the old sages of India; no doubt they cause heat and excitement of mind. But to those who indulge in eating pulses, (grams and other grains which can be divided into two halves) potatoes, sweet potatoes, flesh meat, etc. they are very useful to disinfect their intestinal canal. They are also nervine and brain tonics and are useful in flatulence. Garlic is also a very useful remedy in tuberculosis and worm troubles; it should be eaten raw in moderation with grated cocoanut.

Natural Food or Eliminative Diet.

(1) Select only full ripe or almost ripe fruits in their proper season and fresh vegetables; do not eat over-ripe and also slightly spoiled fruits, faded or wilted vegetables.

(2) Do not eat more than two kinds of fruits or vegetables at a time.

(3) Do not add sugar, salt, pepper or any other ingredient or any condiment to fruits and vegetables; learn to appreciate their natural taste and flavour.

(4) Do not eat any preparations of fruits which are artificially preserved or fruits grown out of their season or preserved in jams, jellies, honey, ete. or in any other way.

(5) Do not boil fruits or vegetables as fire destroys their efficacy and strength-giving qualities such as vitamines, organic matter and organised tissue salts such as phosphates, chlorides, sulphates, etc.

(6) Do not eat dried nuts as they are; soak them previously in pure cold water for several hours say-6 to 12 hours, as the water will revive all their prominent

strength-giving properties. The same rule holds good in all sorts of cereals and grains which are used as human food.

(7) Fruits are useful for those who have a tendency to grow fat; nuts and vegetables are recommended for those who are getting thinner day by day.

(8) Milk may be taken by those who like it but it should be taken fresh as soon as it is squeezed out of the udder.

(9) Ghee, cream, butter, and vegetable oils are avoided the better as they are not natural substances and are bad for the liver; nuts and cereals can supply sufficient fatty or oily substance needed for the body.

(10) Oils, sugar, salt, chillies, spices, fried things, tea, coffee, cocoa, chocolate, liquors, vinegar, wines, tobacco, opium, etc. are avoided the better.

Vitamines

All our food stuffs contain vitamines which are said to be of three varieties A. B. C. Vitamine A is found in milk, nuts and green vegetables, and it is very necessary for the proper growth and sustenance of our bones and teeth. Vitamine B is found in milk, nuts and in all cereals such as wheat, unpolished rice, maize, bajree, millet, beans, pulses, etc. It is very essential for the development of our brains and the nervous system. Vitamine C is found in green vegetables such as cabbages, cauliflower, lettuce, radishes, lady's fingers, spinach, etc. and in some fruits such as peaches, tomatoes, onions, garlic, oranges, sweet limes, lemons, etc.

Though they are in a very minute form in our food stuffs they play an important part in animal economy by supplying our bodies wih vitality and by influencing our ductless glands such as thyroid, the parathyroid the suprarenal, the pineal, the pituitary, the pancreas, the prostate and the testicles.

When our food is cooked these vitamines are burnt away and destroyed by the fire and thus we do not get the real benefit from the food we eat; we eat what is already emasculated, burnt and rendered useless by the fire. Such food becomes tasteless also and to make it tasty we add sea salt, the most objectionable substance, and many other condiments which are nothing but poisons; though they are not able to destroy our life at once they do some harm to our body slowly, steadily but surely

Besides these vitamines, our food stuffs contain some inorganic salts in very minute, atomised, pure and organised form. Though they are in such minute form and in a very small proportion *i. e.* from 2 to 7 percent, without them our bodies will not develop properly and our lives will be extinct sooner than they are meant by Nature. Lower animals die very soon if these salts are removed from their foodstuffs. They are salts of calcium, ferrum (iron), potassium, magnesium, sodium, phosphorus, sulphur, silicon, chlorine, fluorine, iodine, bromine, etc. These, as already mentioned, are in an organised and atomised form in all the food-stuffs and our minute cells are adopted to absorb them in their natural form only. By heating, boiling, cooking and frying our food stuffs we rather injure and destroy the efficacy of these life sustaining substances.

Thereby our food becomes insipid, tasteless and void of strength-giving and life-sustaining properties. Again to improve the taste of the cooked food we add sea-salt which is a very harmful thing. Not satisfied with that too, we add different sorts of condiments which are properly speaking real poisons and mostly all of them are very harmful things. Nature does not want us to partake of any mineral salt direct from earth. She wants us to sustain ourselves from the salts supplied by Her in fruits, nuts and vegetables only. Sea-salt instead of doing good to us does great harm; it causes undue thirst, burning sensation in different parts of the body and generates impurities in the blood which cause itches, neuralgia, cataract and in some rare cases even cancer. Condiments cause flatulence, constipation, sour belching, uric acid troubles, neuralgia, colic, piles, blood-poisoning and so many other diseases as a result of intestinal irregularity. They cause extra salivation first by stimulating them very much to dry them up later on and to cause abnormal thirst.

Those foodstuffs which have a good taste in their natural state can be most easily digested and are also most suited to supply us with vitality as they supply us with vitamines; they are fruits, nuts and milk in fresh and natural form, sugurcane, etc. and also grains before they are dried up, and vegetables which can be eaten raw such as radishes, lettuce, beet root, tomatoes, lady's fingers, etc.

Those foodstuffs which are made fit for eating after being boiled, heated, cooked, steamed, fried, etc. are inferior to natural foods mentioned above, as they lose their vitamines and phosphates during the process of being heated by the fire such as potatoes, all sorts of roots spinach, cabbage, rice, fish, fowl, flesh-meat, etc.

Those food stuffs which are required to be sugared, salted, spiced, pickled, etc. are not suited for the up-keep of health for under that state they become void of their original strength giving properties, do harm by constipating the bowels or causing acidity ; for instance preserves, jams, jellies, pickles, pastries, cakes, fried things, etc. come under that category.

Foods in fluid form such as essences, soups, beverages, cocoa, chocolate, beer, wine, etc. dilate the gastric juice and interfere with the function of digestion and cause liver disorders and constipation, as these are swallowed without being insalivated; they are also not natural.

Dr. Lindlahr says :—

" Every particle of flesh-meat, is as a rule, saturated with the excretion of the cells in the form of uric and other kinds of acids, alkaloids of putrefaction, xanthins, ptomaines, etc. The organism of the meat-eater therefore must dispose not only of cell metabolism, but also of the morbid substances that are already contained in the animal flesh."

6 Duty Assigned by Nature.

Nature wants all her creatures to do their duty. She does not want us to allow our teeth to shirk their work, by making the grinding stones to do their work of grinding, nor does she want the fire to digest our food with boiling, cooking or frying processes. She wants our bodily heat to heat it and digest it well with the help of saliva and gastric juice. We are able to assimilate food and obtain proper nutrition from it when the food is thus digested in a natural way.

The expert engineer of primeval time who designed the grinding stone is the person who laid foundation of our indigestion, dyspepsia, flatulence, stomach-ache, flautlent colic, diarrhoea, tooth-ache, decay and premature fall of teeth, etc. Not being allowed to do their duty our teeth become loose for want of proper exercise and fall off prematurely; such habit is further assisted by the constant touch of sugar, salt and other objectionable substances such as frequent use of very cold drinks and very hot food and drinks. They also become painful and get easily decayed on account of the use of such objectionable substances. Digestion should begin in the mouth in the process of mastication and insalivation. Then only will our stomach find its work of digestion and assimilation of the food rendered easy.

That expert hygienist of old times who devised the method of cooking our food was the prime cause of our dyspepsia, water-brash, scurvy, pyorrhoea and so many other diseases our flesh and blood now-a-days suffer from. The process of cooking devitalizes the food and makes it insipid, indigestible and devoid of health imparting substances; that is why we become weaker and weaker and subject to so many ailments.

That ingenious physician who introduced the use of spices in our daily food is another person who laid foundation of so many diseases from which now a days we suffer. Our saliva, gastric juice, bile, pancreatic juice and chyle have all the necessary substances to digest our natural foodstuffs taken in a proper form. Nature does not want her foodstuffs improved by the addition of sugar, salt, soda, spices, liquors, etc. and her methods changed by devising new artificial plans to help digestion.

(7) Sugar an unnatural and objectionable food.

In the process of refinement the ordinary sugar sold in the market goes through many objectionable and unnatural methods that it loses all the nourishing elements which are found in the sugar-cane and consequently the digestive organs find it difficult to assimilate it properly. For it not only irritates all the digestive organs but even makes our teeth suffer and decay or fall off prematurely.

The teeth of children who eat sugar and sugared substances decay, as a rule, as the sugar irritates the stomach and the teeth sympathise with it. As this sugar is not assimilated by the blood, those who eat much sugar as a rule pass it in their urine, which diseased condition is called Diabetes Mellitus. It also causes worm troubles frequently both among children and grown up persons. It is true that our body requires a supply of sugar every day; but it is not the sugar sold in the bazar. Our body requires sugar from fruits as supplied by Nature in them. Therefore we should consume fruits and not the sugar sold in the bazar as such sugar passes during preparation through objectionable processes which make it unassimilable by our stomach and blood-cells.

The author allows his Diabetic patients to eat freely any fruits in season though they may pass some sugar in their urine for some time ; they are as a rule radically cured of their disease if they abstain from bazar sugar, sea-salt and other unnatural food stuffs, soda, sugared food such as sweetmeats, jams, sugared milk or egg preparations, sweet syrups, etc. These are objectionable and unnatural food-stuffs and they always do harm to the stomach, bowels, urinary organs and also to our teeth and bones; while fruits though they contain sugar are very wholeseme and always do good both to the sick and the healthy as the natural sugar from them is easily assimilated by our blood-cells.

(8) Salt an unnatural and objectionable substance as our food.

Salt whether sea-salt or rock salt is another unwholesome and unnatural substance which we consume daily. Of course our body requires sodium chloride and many other salts. But it does not need such crude and mineral salts. Kind Nature has supplied all the necessary salts in all our foodstuffs and if we partake them fresh as supplied by Her we shall never get ill. For instance the bran and gluten of wheat, rice, maize, millets, bajree and all the cereals contain all the nutritive salts including sodium chloride in their natural and assimilable form. But in our ignorant belief that this husky portion is useless and harmful, we remove it and throw it away and consume only the starchy substance which causes harm to our digestive system.

As we deprive our food-stuffs of these natural salts, we get a craving for sea salt and to satisfy that craving we consume this most objectionable and unnatural substance which does great harm to us. This seasalt is really a poison; if we throw some of it over the ants they die away. If parrots and other birds are made to eat it, they also die sooner or later from its effects. In the human body also, it kills so many living cells; it also preserves in the body all the dead cells which should be eliminated from our body. As it is an unnatural and objectionable stuff Kind Nature tries always to remove it from our body through perspiration, urine and feces. But we consume more and more of it and suffer the consequences.

It not only gives bad smell to our perspiration, urine, and feces but also makes our skin, private parts and anus very foul-smelling. If we leave off eating sea-salt, they will be as clean as all the other organs of the body and even prepuce, labia and armpits will not have any foul smell. It is the dead cells killed by this salt and the non-assimilable bazaar sugar that make them so foul-smelling.

It is over twenty years now that I have been a fruitarian and I subsist on fruits and nuts only. If I feel thirsty I drink cocoanut water or eat a piece of sugarcane or eat some juicy fruit. I find my urine as clear as water and my stools never stink; if they are kept on a piece of paper or on a leaf they dry away but never stink like stools of any other persons, who indulge in fish, fowl, fleshmeat, salted, sugared and cooked food. Any one can make an experiment by leading such a life and find out the truth of this statement.

Besides making our body unclean salt also causes thirst, burning sensation in the body, itches, cataract, constipation or salivation, neuralgia, etc.

Both, sugar and salt kill the living cells and preserve the dead cells; hence naturally and scientifically both are objectionable food-stuffs. My patients suffering from sprue, chronic dysentery or diarrhoea, dropsy, diabetes mellitus, cancer, etc. are much benefited when they abstain from salt and sugar but get worse on the very day they indulge in those unwholesome substances.

(9) Other Objectionable Substances

Aerated waters, tea, coffee, beer, wines, liquors are also very objectionable and unnatural drinks. Saccharine is another very objectionable stuff which doctors generally recommend to their diabetic patients. It often produces cancer and other malignat tumours. Tobacco is another most objectionable substance which is freely indulged in by many persons in these days. In the beginning it increases appetite and removes constipation; but later on it makes the case worse and worse till the person becomes a slave to the habit. It causes dyspepsia, angina pectoris, palpitations of the heart, gastralgia, neuralgic pains in any part of the body, paralysis, vertigo, dimness of sight, blindness, dry cough, asthma, etc.

(10) Fasting.

Fasting in these days has become very popular among some of the Naturopaths who consider it to be the only means of rational and natural cure for all diseases. Of course it is so for the ailments caused by over-eating or caused by errors in diet. Even in such cases, it is not beneficial to fast more than 48 hours; even during this period there is not the least objection to drink water of the tender cocoanuts or to chew sugar-cane-pieces and drink their juice. Fasting for several weeks as recommended by some of the Naturopaths further weakens the constitution of the patient which has already been weakened by disease. Besides, fasting for such long periods is not Natural. Even in the worst cases of indigestion, dyspepsia, acidity, flatulence, fevers, etc. I have not ordered fasting for over 48 hours as there is no need to do so. लंघनं परमौषधम् Fasting is the best medicine Of course, it is so for all those who have comitted errors in their diet. Vitality of the patient is undoubtedly lowered by long fasting. Hence either in acute or chronic ailments such a patient with lowered vitality and decreased activity will not be able to eliminate systemic poisons and waste products from the body though the elimination of such poisons from the body is very necessary both in health and disease.

Animals, wild or domiciled, as a rule do not take any food during illness. Even human beings do not feel any appetite during illness and have no inclination to take any food; they may be getting abnormal thirst due to the inflammation and heat caused by any acute illness but there is no desire for food. But clinging to their daily habits they persist against their inclination in taking food at the suggestion of their relatives and their attending physicians, as they are under the wrong impression that unless food is taken the patients might get weakened and their vitality be decreased. But Nature is the safest guide and neither the healthy nor the sick should take any food when Nature does not call for it that is when they have no appetite and when they have no desire for it. It is not the food taken but the food assimilated that supplies nourishment and the food taken unnecessarily when there is no appetite and the food undigested does, on the contrary, great harm by producing putrefaction and anto-toxin in the body.

Religious fastings of the Jains after sunset till sunrise next day and of the Hindus on Mondays and Thursdays for half a day and on Ekadashees once in a fortnight on the eleventh day after new moon and full moon for the whole day lead to keep them healthy without lowering their vitality in any way.

Such a fast for a short interval assists the body in eliminating wastes and disease products. It gives rest and renewed energy to the digestive organs and corrects defective nutrition.

Fasting for Curative Purpose.

(1) Before commencing a fast the patient should keep his bowels clean by taking the enema daily at least for two or three days; he should also remain on milk and fruits during that period.

(2) During the fast a quick and friction bath should be taken every morning followed by a vigorous towel rub or massage all over the body.

(3) Daily exercise should be taken in proportion to the strength of the patient. Long walks with deep breathing are recommended.

(4) Whenever the patient feels hungry or thirsty a cup of pure water mixed with some fresh fruit juice may be taken. Tender cocoa-nut water or sugar cane juice is preferable.

(5) If the patient feels exhaustion and seems to lose his vitality he can break the fast by taking a cup of fresh milk and an easily digestible fruit. He should not take any hard indigistible food, salt, sugar, etc. at least for a week.

In indigestion, dyspepsia, gastritis, gastralgia, flatulence, flatulent colic, hepatitis, splenitis, enteritis, peritonitis, typhoid fever, dysentery, diarrhœa, sprue, cholera, etc. abstinence from food is very necessary till Nature calls for it. After a prolonged fast great care must be taken in resuming food. Sub-acid fruits such as, sweet limes, oranges, grapes, apples, etc. should be taken first in small quantities, they must be masticated thoroughly and insalivated properly before they are swallowed; juicy vegetables such as lettuce, celery, radishes, cabbages, cauliflower, lady's fingers, etc. may be taken moderately; no spices should be added to them except onions, grated cocoanuts, and fresh lemon juice. The author's experience is that if we eat natural foods properly we are not required to fast for a long period.

A Naturopath should thoroughly aquaint himself with all the properties of every food-stuff and he should be able to instruct his patient what food will suit him and what food will not. He should also be able to know whether sunbath, steambath, shower-bath, enema, bandage, compress, or douche, will suit his patient's case. He should also know what sort of exercise or massage will help him most in eliminating poisons and waste matter from his patients' system. It is Nature that really heals; and the best physician only assists Nature in her healing efforts by helping her to eliminate systemic poison and waste-matter with the help of enema, sunbath, steam-bath, etc. from his patients' body and never thwarts her progress in any way with poisonous drugs, injections, operations, etc.

(11) Advice of a Brahmin to his son During his Thread Ceremony to lead a Natural Life

अंतःपुरनिवासंच छत्रोपानहधारणम् ॥
गवाऽश्वोष्ट्रादियानंच मृदुशय्यांच वर्जय ॥ १ ॥

Translation.—Avoid staying in closed rooms; give up umbrellas and shoes. Avoid riding in vehicles driven by bullocks, horses, camels, etc. and also soft beds.

तैलाभ्यंगंच क्षौरंच गानं नृत्यंच नाटकम् ॥
रात्रौ जागरणं चैव निद्रांच दिवसे त्यज ॥ २ ॥

Translation.—Avoid anointing the body and bathing in hot water. Avoid also shaving, singing, dancing and attending the theatre. Avoid keeping up at nights and sleeping during the day.

सुशीलः स्मितभाषीच मिताहारी तथा भव ॥
लोभमोहानृतं क्रोधं निंदांच परिवर्जय ॥ ३ ॥

Translation.—Be good-natured; smile while you speak. Eat moderately and avoid avarice, greed, falsehood, anger and censure.

प्राणायाम मुषःपानं स्नानं सन्ध्यां क्रमाच्चर ॥
पश्चात्सूर्यमुपस्थाय वेदाध्ययनमाचर ॥ ४ ॥

Translation.—Early in the morning take breathing exercise and drink a cupful of pure cold water; then bathe and perform *Sandhya* meditation; afterwards salute the sun and read *vedas.*

त्यक्त्वाऽत्यम्लकटुक्षारमातितिक्तं कषायकम् ॥
युक्ताहारविहारैश्च योगाभ्यासं समाचर ॥ ५ ॥

Translation.—Avoid, very sour, pungent, saltish bitter and astringent foods; take wholesome food and proper exercise and practise *yoga* philosophy.

क्षीरगोधूमनीवारैः कंदमूलफलैस्तथा ॥
मधुरं लघुपाकंच नित्यं भोजनमाचर ॥ ६ ॥

Translation.—Eat daily tasty food which can be easily digested such as milk, wheat, millet (Neewar), roots, vegetables and fruits.

मत्स्यं मांसंच मद्यंच रुक्षाहारंच वर्जय ॥
वीर्यं संरक्ष्य यत्नेन स्वयं भव जितेंद्रियः ॥ ७ ॥

Translation.—Avoid fish, flesh, liquor, and all objectionable food. Preserve your semen assiduously; avoid its waste and control your passions.

कुरुष्व सततं कर्म स्वधर्मं परिपालय ॥
एवं द्वादशवर्षाणि ब्रह्मचर्यं समाचर ॥ ८ ॥

Translation,—Do your duty; obey your religious dictates. Thus observe celibacy for the next 12 years.

As a rule a Brahamin celebrates the Thread Ceremany of his son when he attains his eighth year long before he finishes his eleventh year and he is supposed to observe celibacy for 12 years and lead a natural life advised above and lead a married life there after.

(12) Natural Mode of Life and Longevity.

The Natural mode of living not only confers immunity from disease but also ensures a long and a healthy life. The lion known as the king of beasts and the tiger, match to the lion in strength, feed on raw flesh; but they live about 25 years only; while some African apes such as chempanzies and gorillas who feed on raw fruits and nuts are more than a match for the lion and the tiger in strength and stratagem; further they live for more than 200 years; they also possess strength enough to easily bend and break to pieces the heaviest of the guns of the lion and ape-hunters. Men who lead a natural life and subsist on fruits, nuts and vegetables lead a hearty and healthy life and live more than a century. Democritus and Hippocrates the Greek naturalists lived one hundred and nine years of a happy and joyous life without any illness. The Sweedish veteran Mittelsted who during his military career of 67 years had fought in 17 battles and who led mostly a natural life lived 112 years without any illness. Effingham, our

English soldier who subsisted mostly on milk, fruits and nuts died at the ripe age of 144 years. Thomas Parr lived 152 years; he used to subsist on milk and fruits and was always in good health. King Charles heard of him, sent for him, and in order to do him honour had a splendid repast set before him. This caused his death for the post mortem examination showed that it was due to disturbed digestion while both of his internal and external organs were in good condition.

The Norwegian Drakenberg died at the age of 146. Joseph Surringtion died at the age of 150. The Hungarian Bowin died in 1750 at the ripe age of 172. Another authentic instance may be mentioned of a Russian veteran who was born in 1623 and died in 1825 aged 202. (Herald of Health Aug. 1920).

In the records of St. Leonard's Church, London, there may be seen an entry of a birth and death which one might be tempted to doubt if it were not invested with full official authority, that of Thomas Carn born January 25, 1588 and died 1795 aged 207 years; he saw 12 sovereigns occupying the British throne.

People of one hundred years of age and upwards are by no means rare in the rural population of the Herzegovina, and there are some villages in the mountain districts of that country in which it very rarely happens that an inhabitant dies before the age of eighty. A peasant named Anton Turitsch had attained the age of 130 and was living in a healthy state in 1920. (Herald of Health August 1920).

Ivan Kusmin a peasant aged 138 years was admitted into the Obuchow hospital in St. Petersburg on the 3rd October 1895 John Saveire de Limo died in 1730 at the age of 198. Peter Maffens mentions in his History of India a man named Numisde Cogua who died in 1556 aged 370 years. His teeth beard and hair grew four times. (Herald of Health Aug. 1928) Bheeshma lived over 177 years. Ashwatthama, Balee, Vyasa, Hanumantha, Vibheeshana, Kripa and Parashurama are said to be the longest lived in India. They are known as *chiranjeevis i. e.*, the Longest-lived.

अश्वत्थामा बलिर्व्यासो मारुतिश्च विभीषणः
कृपः परशुरामश्च सप्तैते चिरंजीविनः

This shows that among human beings those who lead natural life can live over a century free from disease.

Why then does a man die early? Why does he suffer from so many ailments? It is because he eats too much, drinks too much and consumes unnatural substances and makes use of so many non-nutritious unwholesome, and poisonous substances. Will not a candle last less time if it is burnt at both ends or if it is exposed to strong winds, dust, butter-flies, etc.? Man breathes less and breathes in an unnatural way by over-burdening his stomach; he eats more, he drinks more and as a result he purges more and he urinates more than he should do; he also makes use of so many stimulants, narcotics, and so many poisonous substances. This being so, is there any cause for wonder that he suffers from so many diseases and dies prematurely?

The more we over-burden our stomach and over-tax our liver with tea, coffee, alcohol, salt, sugar, flesh-food spiced food, fried things, oily substances, cheese, butter, ghee, pickles, preserved foods and so many other unnatural unwholesome and artificially prepared dainties the more dyspeptic we shall be and loss of appetite or voracious appetite, flatulence, constipation, acidity, debility, etc., will be the result. These ailments being very common look very trifling but they lay the foundation of more serious complaints such as gastric or enteric fever, biliousness or jaundice, enlargement or cirrhosis of liver, hepatic or intestinal colic, gall or renal stones, hepatitis or splenitis, enteritis or appendicitis, diarrhoea or dysentery, scurvy or pyorrhoea, diabetes insipidus or mellitus, tuber-culosis of lungs or bowels, ulcer or cancer of the liver, etc., etc. All these diseases and also so many other ailments to which we are subject are the consequences of our own transgressions of the laws of Nature. We devise so many unnatural methods to cure all the diseases but we fail. If we cure one disease another, a graver one, follows it! Therefore the best way to be free from ailments is to return to Nature and obey her laws which alone will enable us to lead a healthy and a happy life.

CHAPTER XII

Natural and Rational Treatment of Diseases: Hints to the physicians.

(1) The cause of any disease is the violation of Nature's laws for instance (*a*) breathing through the mouth instead of nostrils, inhaling foul air loaded with effluvia, nicotine, etc. (*b*) drinking impure water, stimulating beverages, aerated waters, or alcoholic drinks (*c*) eating flesh-meat and other food not meant by Nature for human cousumption. (*d*) wearing improper dress for instance corsets, high heeled or tight boots, multiplicity of clothes so as to impede fresh air from touching the skin (*e*) untimely sleep, (*f*) lack of proper exercise (*g*) love-less marriages among blood relations such as cousins, etc. sensuality, sexual wrongs, dissipation (*h*) immoral thoughts, fear, worry, etc. contribute partly or wholly to the cause of disease and degeneration.

(2) When faulty habits of living have clogged the system and do not allow the body to perform its functions properly, Nature tries to free the system from those impurities by some acute diseases, the suppression of which with drugs makes them assume other forms or turn them into chronic and so called incurable diseases.

(3) In these days of rapid medical progress innumerable poisons, coal tar preparations, vaccines, serums, injections of different nature, etc. have been devised to suppress diseases immediately. But all these serve as extra foreign substances or poisons in the body and sooner or later produce some obstinate or so called incurable disease.

(4) Naturopathy can cure all diseases. It can cure not only acute and chronic diseases but even the so called obstinate and incurable ones by expelling from the body all foreign matter or impurities which are the main cause of disease. A Naturopath knows that it is Nature that heals and all that he should do is to aid her in her healing process which consists of elimination of poisons from the body by purifying the blood.

(5) Physicians are attempting to cure anaemia with crude iron preparations, acidity of the stomach with sodium, glandular troubles with iodine, itches with sulphur and zinc ointments, rickets with lime water, etc. This mode of treatment is not in accordance with the laws of Nature and is most objectionable as it checks the trouble and makes the case worse later on by changing the symptoms of the disease. Nature wants all animals to be fed with vegetable substances only; she also wants their ailments to be cured with her bounties. And for this purpose the uninverse abounds with her bounties.

Nature's Bounties

Fresh Air:—

(1) A plentiful supply of fresh air is very necessary both in health and disease.

(2) Exposure of the whole body to fresh air stimulates the skin and makes the pores work properly. They inhale oxygen and lighten the burden of the work lungs are required to do, they also help kidneys by bringing out proper perspiration.

(3) Loose white thin garments are the proper dress to allow the fresh air to touch the skin freely.

(4) Inhale pure fresh air; take deep breaths through the nostrils only and not through the month.

Pure Water

(1) Pure cold water should be used for daily ablutions and therapeutical applications.

(2) Neither ice nor hot water applications should be used in fevers, inflammations and congestions.

(3) Length of time and mode of application should be determined by an experienced Hydropath to suit the condition of the patient.

(4) If the patient cannot bear cold water, neutral water may be used till he is able to bear cold applications. (See Scientific Hydropathy.)

3 Sunlight

(1) The whole body should be exposed to sunlight whenever convenient.

(2) If the whole body cannot be exposed, the ailing limb or the ailing part of the body should be given sun bath so long as the patient can bear the sun.

(3) If the patient can't bear hot sun he should begin with the mild sun gradually increasing the time of exposure and brightness of the sun until he is able to bear the midday sun and until he perspires freely.

(4) The patient should keep up the habit of taking the sun-bath even after the cure. If he cannot take it daily he may take it occasionally whenever convenient.

4 Diet

(1) Both in health and in disease no food should be taken unless one feels hungry and gets the desire to eat.

(2) Only the food supplied by Nature should be taken and it should be masticated throughly and insalivated properly before it is allowed to pass into the stomach.

(3) In indigestion, dyspepsia, flatulent colic and febrile conditions fasting till the patient feels an appetite is to be observed very strictly.

(4) However a little fruit juice diluted or undiluted may be given to allay thirst.

Treatment.

Abdomen bloated :—Tepid enema, massage, fasting till the patient feels hungry; light food such as fruits, milk, conjee, etc.; avoid flesh-meat and pulses.

Abdominal Colic :—Fomentation with heated sand. In obstinate cases tepid enema and massage. For diet see Abdomen bloated.

Abscess :—An inflamed painful surface of the skin. Fomentation for 30 minutes or sun bath as long as can be born by the patient. Then a warm compress with a piece of dry flannel over it. If warm compress can not be born, Hot Shower both. Diet—fruits, milk and whole meal wheat bread. Avoid fleshmeat and pulses.

Acidity, sour belching :—Fasting till hunger calls for food. Enema. Easily digestible food. A cup of cold water early in the morning; walking exercise after it.

Adenitis, inflammation of glands—Sun bath; Massage and cold compress with dry flannel over it.

After-pains, pains that follow delivery—Fomentations with heated sand; Massage.

Ague, Malarial or intermittent fever—Sunbath or steambath during chill or shivering stage; Neptune's Girdle or cold compress during hot stage. Neutral enema every day if bowels do not work properly. Avoid fried food and cold substances such as curds, butter milk, cold drink, etc.

Albuminuria, passing of albumin in the urine—Hip-bath. Diet-milk and fruits.

Alcoholism—Shower bath; cold compress over the abdomen. Diet—sour fruits and butter milk.

Amenorrhoea, absence of menses—Hot foot bath every night at bed time. If obstinate cold Hip-bath also in the morning followed by light exercise.

Anaemia, poverty of blood—Hip bath followed by brisk walk in the bright sun. Eat-red coloured fruits and vegetables freely.

Aneurism, a blood tumor—shower bath; enema; Diet—milk and fruits,

Angina Pectoris; spasm of the chest—Fomentation; hot foot bath; Enema daily. Diet—milk and fruits.

Apoplexy, rush of blood to the head caused by heaty food, stimulating drinks, stroke of lightning or sunstroke—Make the patient lie with head on a high cushion; loosen his dress and give an air-bath at once; give a tea-spoonful of fresh water frequently; shower, bath and massage over his neck and spine. Neutral enema; Neutral bath; milk and fruit diet.

Appendicitis, Inflammation of appendix—the symptoms are constipation furred tongue, vomiting, fever and sudden pain at first over the whole abdomen which afterwards localises to the right iliac fossa—The causes are improper or unnatural diet. In less than one per cent of cases however, seeds and other foreign bodies are found located in the appendix. Dr. Lindlahr says—"Appendicitis is practically always preceded by an inactive, atrophic condition of the intestines which favours the accumulation of fecal matter in the caecum and descending colon which in turn leads to inflammation of the caecum and appendix.

Dr. Lindlahr M. D. in his philosophy of natural cure says:—

"Says the surgeon, if it is appendicitis only an opertion will save the patient's life". This we positively deny and have proved untrue in hundreds of cases. We have never had an operation for appendicitis performed on one of our patients and we have not lost a single case. Our own records and our reports to the Board of Health attest this fact. If our diagnosis be questioned I answer that we have taken numerous cases which had already been treated for appendicitis by other physicians who claimed that operation was absolutely necessary.

"Several years ago a member of the French Academy of science published statistics showing that appendicitis in different countries and in different classes of society increases in exact ratio with the consumption of meat. The principal causes of constipation and there-fore of appendicitis are meat, fish, fowl, eggs, coffee, and white bread. Flesh foods taken in excess result in putrefaction; this favours constipation, the development of bacteria, inflammation and later on diarrhoea which are followed gradually by atony and atrophy.

The treatment for acute appendicitis is the same as that for any other acute inflammatory feverish disease. The essentials are plenty of fresh air, absolute fasting, hydrotherapy and manipulative treatment. Massage and water compresses with milk and fruit juice whenever the patients are hungry have cured many cases radically. Enema is very necessary for constipation.

Appetite depraved, craving for earth, chalk, charcoal, salt, salted fish or meat, etc. is due to errors in diet only—Avoid all unnatural food; take milk, fruits, nuts, whole meal bread, etc.; remove constipation by the regular use of enema. *Appetite* lost or voracious is also the result of improper diet—treat the patients in the same way.

Arterio-sclerosis, hardening of arterial walls—Shower bath. Sunbath and Hot-foot bath at bed-time. Milk and fruit diet. Avoid tobacco, liquor, fleshmeat, tea, coffee and aerated waters.

Arthritis, inflammation of joints caused by exposure or uric acid troubles—Massages, sunbath, shower bath, douche-bath. cold water compress over which a piece of dry flannel is to be tied; whole meal wheat bread, milk and fruits recommended. Avoid fish, foul, flesh-meat, pulses, potatoes, sweet potatoes and all wind-producing and uric acid producing substances; use an enema early in the morning to keep the bowels clean.

Asthma,—Enema daily; fasting occasionally. In obstinate cases hip-bath, milk and fruit diet. Fasting every night. See Scientific Hydropathy.

Atrophy, the wasting of any organ—shower bath, sun bath; wholemeal wheat bread, milk and fruits.

Back-ache—Enema and Massage

Baldness—Shower baths and Sunbaths

Bedsores—Water compress, sunbaths.

Belching—Enema, fastiug till the patient feels hungry, light diet.

Biliousness—Light diet; a cup of cold water morning and at bedtime.

Bites—of poisonous animals—see poisonous bites.

Boil—treat like Abscess.

Bone, curvature of—Massage, shower bath; sunbath; milk and fruit diet.

Bone fractured—cold water compress over which a piece of dry flannel should be used as bandage renewing when it gets dry; whole meal wheat bread, milk and fruit diet.

Brainfag—Shower bath and sunbath

Breath offensive—Enema, fruits and milk diet.

Bronchitis—Breathing exercise; cold water frictions to the chest; sunbath; enema when constipated.

Bruises—Water compress; sunbath.

Burns and Scalds—sunbath ; compress of warm water.

Cancer is a malignant tumour formed chiefly of epithelial cells. It is caused by abnormal vitiation of blood, and lymph and generally occurs in persons of *psoric* constitution who lead an unnatural life and cause vitiation of blood grossly. It may appear on the eye, nose, lip, tongue, tonsil, breast, ovary, uterus, stomach, liver, spleen, intestines, kidneys, glans, genitals, testicles, labia and in any lymphatic gland. It has three stages (1) a closed hard tumour without pain (2) painful tumour which begins to ulcerate (3) cancerous sore with thin serous discharge at first bloody and later on purulent and offensive. It causes darting lacerating or lancinating pain and distroys surrounding tissues and makes the life of the patient very miserable till death intervenes.

Sir william Banks, an eminent British physician declares that the most numerous victims of cancer are high livers, flesh-meat eaters and coffee and alcohol-drinkers. Dr. Senn says—"It is where eating is made an art that cancer is most prevalent" "Drinking, gourmandising and all unnatural habits of women help to plant the seeds of cancer"

Prof. Bell says:—Smoking plays a large part in the production of a pre-cancerous state". The primary and predisposing cause of cancer is a vitiated blood stream produced by the effects of flesh food".

In about 200 cases of cancer which the author had occasion to see and watch, he observed that they were chiefly among tobacco-smokers, tobacco-eaters, opium-eaters, chunam-eaters, salted fish-eaters, salted meat-eaters, frequent flesh-meat eaters, excessive salt and pickle-eaters, and those who make frequent use of aerated waters, saccharine and other tar-products, and also those addicted to alcohol, sexual sinners and those who suffered long from constipation. All the female patients had scanty and irregular menses and both male and female patients were of psoric constitution. Many of these had been vaccinated several times or had prophylactic injections for plague, typhoid, tuberculosis, or cholera. There were also some cases among those who had got their teeth removed on account of pyorrhoea.

" Schweninger, a prominent European (Allopathic) physician says :—" The Radium treatment is a gigantic swindle. Others claim to have produced, within forty eight hours, most marvellous cures of cancer by means of the radium rays. The surgeons declare that there may be some good in the radium treatment, but that, after all, the safest way lies in the early removal of tumours by the knife. About ten years ago similar positive and extravagant claims were made for the Roentgen-rays. Institutions for X ray treatment sprang up all over the country but what has been the result ? It is now a well established fact that the X-rays instead of curing cancer, create it. Already evidence is accumlating which indicates that the radium emanations are just as dangerous as the X-rays. These agents, on account of immense vibratory velocity and power are altogether too strong and too destructive for the tissues of the human body. I have over thirty newspaper clippings gathered during the last ten years which report the development of cancer-like growths after exposure to X-rays. The radium rays are more powerful than the X-rays." (Lindlahr). Radium and X-ray can cure cancer only when administered in Homoeopathic high potencies according to symptoms.

Drugs, knife, X Rays, Radium treatment, etc. have not cured a single case of cancer entirely as yet; all doctors and medical authors admit that there is no treatment for cancers. They say that they cannot be cured by medicine and they must be operated upon; but they always recur after extirpation." The author has cured several cases of cancer with Homeopathic medicines according to the symptoms with fruit and milk diet. Salt, sugur, tobacco, liquor, flesh-meat, fish, fowl, pickles, condiments, tea, coffee, saccharine and all unnatural substances were asked to be avoided and the patients had no recurrence. The natural methods tried were sunbath direct and through blue and green glasses. Hib-bath with friction to the lower part of the abdomen and compresses both hydropathic and homeopathic with suitable drugs according to homeopathic principles; enema whenever constipated, etc.

Cancer: Mrs. S. wife of a butcher of Rudnitz, Leipsic had tried every possible remedy for her serious disorder, namely cancer of the breast and nose, but all in vain. She was in a deplorable condition. On the breast there was a deep sore putrescent and corroding, and so large that it could scarcely be covered by the hand. Half the nose was already destroyed and on the forehead two large red cancerous tumours had formed which were on the point of breaking. After examination I gave necessary directions for the treatment which pròved most successful. First the tumours on the forehead disappeared; then the breast healed and finally the nose in 9 months. Today she is again a good-looking woman. This miracle, for so it must seem to all who had seen this patient during the worst period of the disease was worked simply by means of natural diet, hip and sitz-baths and profuse perspiration without any local treatment whatever, whether of the breast, nose or forehead (Kuhne).

Cancer of the lip. An old gentleman 72 years of age had been treated for six years by the most famous Allopaths and Homeopaths for cancer of lip. The growths on the lip continually developed and there was a troublesome and perpetual flow of saliva. I diagnosed the patient and found that the encumbrance had risen more from the front and sides toward the head. The result of my treatment was soon to be remarked. Already on the first day the disagreeable salivation ceased and the new growths, proliferations and open wounds began to diminish. Within ten days the latter had healed up and the lip was now but one third its former size. In eleven days the patient had attained the result which the former six years treatment had not been able to produce. Here is a case of curing cancer which the medical profession, as is well known, declares to be impossible (Kuhne).

Carbuncle is a large boil with terrible burning pain discharging pus from several openings; persons of decreased vitality, chiefly diabetic patients suffer from it. Treatment—cold water bandages and sunbaths. Milk, fruits, nuts and wholemeal bread are recommended; bowels must be kept regularly moved with the use of enema. In obstinate cases one or two steambaths weekly and one or two hip-baths daily.

Caries of bone, molecular decay of bone—sunbath and hip-bath daily. Steam bath twice a week; enema daily; milk, fruits, nuts and wholemeal bread without salt and sugar.

Chancres are of two sorts; they appear as swellings on the sexnal organs after intercourse with diseased person. Hard chancre, the primary symptom of syphilis permeates the whole body with its poison, while soft chancre is a local disease. A very slight wound or fissure of the skin is sufficient to admit its infection; the incubation lasts about thirty to thirty six hours; the part itches and becomes red and in 48 hours forms a chancre in which pus forms on the fourth day. It then bursts and festers and gradually spreads around or only downwards where the tissues get rotten. As a rule there are several at a time which unite and become one large abscess. In mild cases the abscess heals in four to six weeks; if special care is taken it heals in three. In neglected cases from exertion bubo arises in the groin; in the third week it may burst. It may take several weeks to heal completely. Treatment—take a piece of lint, dip it in pure water previously well boiled and brought to the temperature of about 75 and lay it on the swollen place with a piece of linen four folded; wrap it up in clean flannel; this must be changed four to six times a day. If the lint sticks to the wound, fully wet it with pure tepid water before trying to remove it,—give 2 or 3 hip baths daily; keep compress in the groins to prevent buboes and ask the patient not to exert much; vapour baths may be needed twice or thrice a week. The diet should be mild and non-stimulating, such as milk and fruits; bowels must be kept clean daily with enema; coffee, tea, liquor, tobacco and meat should be avoided.

The author has treated more than half a dozen cases of chancres with green-water bandages and sun-bath (rays being reflected through green glass). Enema daily; fruit and milk diet recommended; the sores washed clean with soap-nut-water.

Chicken-pox—see zymotic diseases.

Chlorosis or green sickness is so named from the greenish pale colour of the skin which the patients develop during the illness; as a rule girls from the age of 16 to 25 are subject to it. The causes are wrong diet, use of condiments, too much salt, tobacco, coffee and other narcotics, lack of exercise, living in ill-ventilated houses, sexual abuse, irregular menses, etc. The symptoms are disorders of the digestive organs such as voracious appetite or want of appetite, bad taste in the mouth, constipation, vomiting, abdominal pains, scanty urine, pains in the head and back, coldness of extremeties, chilly sensation all over the body, etc. The treatment should be long walks in the bright sun, air baths, sunbaths and hip-baths daily; breathing exercise oxygenates the blood and imparts rosy colour to the cheeks and healthy colour to the skin. Diet should be natural; milk fruits, nuts and fresh vegetables should be taken freely. Enema should be used whenever bowels are constipated. All stimulating drinks and narcotics must be avoided. The mind must me kept cheerful in good company and bad habits (sexual wrongs) should be put a stop to.

Cholera Infantum, cholera morbus, diarrhoea and dysentery with bloody or slimy motions should be treated with light diet, if possible with fasting. If the patient is too weak and can not fast, a little milk not heated on strong fire but heated by keeping the cup of milk in boiling water may be given in small quantities; if the patient feels thirsty a little pure water with pomegranate juice may be given. After the cure, great care must be observed in breaking the fast; the patient may feel abnormal hunger but light food must be supplied in the beginning in moderation; enema may be used to wash the colon clean; sunbath directly on the abdomen may produce very satisfactory results.

Cholera Asiatica—The author could not get an opportunity to treat cases of cholera asiatica with nature's bounties as the patient's relatives could not trust in the natural treatment of cholera and asked for Homeopathic Medicines only. See Practical Chromopathy and

Scientific Hydropathy by the author for the treatment. For Homeopathic treatment see Homeopathic Self-help.

Chorea—see nervous diseases.

Cold—Enema daily of neutral water (99). and sun-baths twice or thrice a day will cure even the most obstinate colds. In obstinate cases *a steam bath* will abort it soon. If a person catches cold frequently the best way of curing that tendency is to accustom to cold baths and cold water drinking; enema is to be used whenever bowels are constipated and sunbath to be taken twice daily. These cold water baths inure the patient against catching cold frequently.

Congestion, abnormal accumulation of blood in any part of the body. It may be in the head, chest, liver, kidneys, etc. Treatment–Showerbath and massage. Hot foot bath at bed time and non-stimulating diet.

Constipation is the prime cause of nearly ninety percent of diseases. In these days people who lead an unnatural, luxurious and fashionable life first suffer from constipation; by neglecting it they suffer from many other diseases. Tea, coffee, cocoa, and other beverages, aerated waters, especially those which are prepared with saccharine, wines, liquors, white bread, toasts, biscuits, lozenges, ice-cream, pudding, cheese, cakes, fried preparations, salt, sugar, spices, condiments, pickles, jams, *papads*, chutneys and other preserved foods, fish, foul, fleshmeat, tobacco and other narcotics all contribute to produce constipation. Rice, white bread and other starchy food stuffs which are deprived of their natural salts also cause constipation.

In our stomach and bowels these food stuffs turn into a sticky substance like book-binder's paste and stick in the inner portion of our bowels and not being easily evacuated cause constipation.—Change of diet is very necessary. Wholemeal bread prepared from wheat, oats, maize or rice, fruits in season chiefly yellow coloured ones with a cup of pure water morning and bedtime will cure even the most obstinate cases of constipation; enema may be required to be used for some days till the liver begins to work properly.

Severe constipation—Mrs. F. wife of a doctor of A. had suffered for about 20 years from severe constipation. Every remedy had failed. When she came to consult me she stated that after all her experience she really had no hope of being cured. Natural diet improved her in a week and all her complaints disappeared completely in a short time (Kuhne).

Consumption of *lungs* now known as phthisis pulmonalis and consumption of *bowels* known as tabes mesenterica are caused by gross disobedience to the laws of Nature and they can be cured by obeying Nature only. In both diseases, the blood gets vitiated and tubercles are formed. When developed they cause cough in the former while they cause foul diarrhoea in the latter. In both diseases the patient first overburdens his stomach with unnatural food taken in large quantities which as a rule over-taxes the liver and causes engorgement of the colon. The stomach being over loaded, the patient breathes through the mouth instead of through the nostrils or breathes imperfectly through the nose only. Thereby the lungs do not get oxidised properly and tubercles arise in one of them or in both of them. Engorged colon as a rule debilitates the bowels and vitiates the blood by the re-absorption of fecal matter accumulated there and as a result tubercles are formed there. The food not being digested and assimilated properly causes diarrhoea first of undigested matter and later on of foul rotten food and of the substances of the tubercles themselves. Hectic fever and exhausting sweats are present as a rule.

Cold water compress with a bandage of dry flannel over the affected region, sunbath and hip-bath followed by brisk walk in sunlight; natural diet chiefly containing fresh milk, fruits in season and whole-meal bread; enema whenever constipated. In most obstinate cases if the patient has sufficient vitality but does not get perspired after taking sunbath, steambath once or twice a week followed by hip-bath and a brisk walk. Tobacco, spices flesh-meat and liquor should be avoided. If the patient has sufficient vitality he should try exercises for the development of chest mentioned in chapter IX.

Cough :—See Respiratory organs

Croup :—See Respiratory organs

Cystitis, Inflammation of the bladder—Hip-bath and shower-bath daily. Cold water massage; enema early in the morning or at betime. Diet--milk, fruits, whole meal bread. Avoid salt tobacco, liquor and spices.

Deafness :—Shower bath followed by massage over the region of the ears. Hip-bath followed by sunbath and brisk walk. Natural diet. See colour treatment in Practical Chromopathy.

Diabetes Insipidus :—Consists in the excess of urine without an increase of sugar in it. Shower bath and sunbath over the region of kidneys. In obstinate cases brisk walks in the sun to induce perspiration after a hip-bath. Easily digestible food. Enema whenever the least constipation is noticed.

Diabetes Mellitus :—is characterised by an increase of sugar in the urine. Really speaking, Diabetes mellitus does not consist in passing sugar in the urine but in the non-assimilation of sugar from the food we eat. Our system requires sugar but not that bazar sugar which is prepared by heating the sugar-cane-juice for a length of time in an artificial way. It can only assimilate sugar from sweet fruits and starchy food. Our allopathic brethren can show wonderful decrease of sugar in the urine by making the patient avoid all fruits and all starchy food, and take saccharine in his tea and other preparations, but the system is starved for want of natural sugar so much needed and the patient gets emaciation and goes to an early grave; or his blood gets vitiated from the use of saccharine and sooner or later suffers from cancer or other malignant diseases. The best course is therefore to allow the patient to eat fruits and starchy food which is natural and ask him to avoid saccharine and bazar sugar entirely. This will not reduce the sugar in urine at once but it will build up his health so well that he will be able to assimilate the sugar properly from the fruits and starch and there will be radical cure of the complaint without any unpleasant symptoms of the disease. Enema should be used daily to clear the bowels. Sunbaths should be taken daily to induce perspiration; sugar, salt, condiments, liquor, coffee, tobacco, fleshmeat, fowl, fish, pickles, etc. should be avoided. In obstinate cases hip-baths and sunbaths Should be taken. Long walks morning and evening; massages over the region of liver and kidneys.

" Medical science prescribes an almost exclusive meat diet for diabetic patients; but in this way diabetes is not known to have been cured. This disease is like others a consequence of an unnatural mode of life and can therefore only be cured by a strictly natural life." (A. Just). The author recommends peaches, jambuls, pomegranets, plantains, caryca papaya, and all fruits in season; cocoanut, *sesamum*, almonds, pistachio and other nuts, cereals before they are dried up and in some cases wholemeal bread and milk also.

Diarrhoea and **dysentery** are caused by errors in diet. They should be treated by regulating the diet with the use of enema to cleanse the bowels. In obstinate cases the patients should fast till they feel hungry. To break the fast keep the patients on fruits, milk and pomegranet juice only. Several obstinate cases have yielded satisfactorily to the above treatment combined with sun-bath over the abdomen.

Diarrhoea and dysentery:—Mrs. W. an American lady complained of dysentery and chronic diarrhoea which had been going on for 4 years the remedies she had tried at the advice of numerous physicians proved quite ineffectual. I prescribed easily digestible diet suited to her condition, cooling friction baths thrice a day and thrice steam baths each week. Her troubles disappeared after 3 week's treatment. (Kuhne).

Dyspepsia also is caused by errors in diet. Some people eat beyond their capacity to digest, others eat indigestible food, some others swallow their food without masticating and insalivating it. Is it any wonder if they suffer from indigestion and dyspepsia? If the ailment is caused by errors in diet it is quite plain that it will be cured by regulating the diet only. Milk, fruits and easily digestible food properly masticated and insalivated will improve the condition of the patient steadily and surely; occasional fasting from 24 to 48 hours, walking exercise, removal of constipation with enema may also be required in obstinate cases.

Ear-ache:—Foment the region of the ear with hot sand or a sponge or towel dipped in hot water.

Ear-discharge:—Syringe the ear with tepid water, but take care that the stream does not touch the drum but touches the sides only. In obstinate cases use an enema to cleanse the bowels; avoid all wind producing substances, condiments and all heaty food.

" **Deafness and Dumbness due to Congestion of the brain**:—Four year old girl of Mrs. S. of L. was deaf and dumb, as the result of vaccination. The mother said numerous medical applications had proved of no avail. The poor child had been severely maltreated by means of operations and corrosives and used to cry whenever it saw a physician; on account of its crying and fear I could not thoroughly examine her. However friction baths, natural diet, plenty of exercise in the fresh sunny air improved her in two weeks and she became all right in 6 weaks, she could hear and speak and was not shy (Kuhne).

Eczema :—See skin diseases

Enteric Fever :—See fevers

Enteritis :—See inflammation

Epilepsy :—See nervous diseases

Erysipelas :—See zymotic diseases

Eyes:—For all eye troubles caused by over-strain or injury use eye wash as follows : Submerge the whole head in pure cold water (but not too cold to cause u easiness) and open the lids and shake the head to and fro six times. Repeat the process thrice a day. Expose the eyes then to the mild sun; if you cannot do so, slowly rub the region of the eyes to create warmth by quickening the circulation.

In all constitutional eye diseases try the same method of treatment and take the greatest care to keep the bowels regular by making free use of enema even twice a day if necessary. Special attention should be paid to diet; only natural food stuffs must be allowed ; all the heaty food stuffs, condiments, salted food, tea, coffee and other stimulating drinks, tobacco, opium, hemp and other injurious substances should be avoided.

In granulations, cataract, glaucoma, syphilitic iritis, hypopyon and other obstinate diseases even salt, sugar, and chillies should be avoided.

Rules for Preserving and Improving Eyesight.

(1) Don't enter a dark room at once

(2) Don't expose your eyes at once to the bright sun as soon as you come out of a dark room.

(3) Avoid dark rooms as much as possible during day time.

(4) Dont read in twilight.

(5) Dont read in a lying posture.

(6) Dont read while driving in a car.

(7) Dont read faint or small type

(8) If you are reading before a lamp keep a plate filled in with cold water near you, between the lamp and your eyes.

(9) If you are using a kerosine oil lamp use a blue chimney over it and if you are using electric light use blue bulb.

(10) After reading much or straining your eyes refresh them by laving them in cool pure water or by exposing them to cool fresh air.

Fever is Nature's effort to remove foreign substances from the system by burning it off or by expelling it through the pores, by inducing perspiration; therefore it should not be checked by strong doses of aspirin or phenacetin but watched and moderated when it becomes dangerously high and prevented when the temperature returns to the normal.

In all chronic diseases where the fever is entirely absent, our effort should be to bring on fever and sustain it for some time. The process of inducing perspiration and cleaning the bowels with enema must be the means to expel foreign matter from the system and to keep the patient on natural diet and on natural mode of living. In such cases we must have recourse to fresh air, pure water, bright sunlight, proper rest and sleep, proper exercise and natural diet.

Catarrhal fever, ephemeral fever caused by indigestion, injury, exposure, or suppression of perspiration, etc., intermittent fever, ague, malarial fever caused by drinking stagnant water or mosquito bite or by staying near dirty ditches or gutters, or staying in jungles (forests), camp fever, ghat fever, remittent fever, hay fever, typhoid fever, typhus, scarlet or yellow fevers, Bubonic plague, etc. are all the result of Nature's burning the foreign matter in the system hence they should not be suppressed with drugs or injections or with coal tar preparations. Sun-bath during the cold stage, and Neptune's girdle during hot stage are the best measures. Enema for constipation. Massages in case of liver and spleen enlargements are also necessary. Breathing exercise and non-stimulating, light diet are also needed—See Scientific Hydropathy by the author.

Gall-stones are caused by liver disorders:—Avoid fatty substances, fried things and chiefly flesh-meat and pulses. Keep the patient strictly on milk and fruits ; conjee, prepared from rice, wheat, oats or maize may be taken moderately ; massage all over the region of liver ; give in obstinate cases hip-baths daily followed with brisk walks. Enema should be given whenever bowels are constipated.

Gastritis is the result of errors in diet—avoid all heaty food; milk, fruits, nuts, conjee prepared from rice, wheat, maize or oats may be given moderately; do not give hot or cold food, avoid tobacco, tea, coffee liquor, pickles, and condiments.

German measles:—See zymotic diseases

Glands:—Adenoids, tonsillitis, mumps, goitre, scrofula, enlargement of prostate and all glandular troubles should be treated with massage, sun-baths, and compresses. Enema and light non-stimulating diet are also very necessary.

Gonorrhoea and gleet. Gonorrhoea is urethritis causing discharge of pus. It is caused by sexual intercourse with a person suffering from that disease. Gleet is the chronic condition of Gonorrhoea :—Use syringes of water exposed to the sunlight by keeping it in a green bottle ; drink the same water, one ounce twice a day morning and at bedtime ; avoid all heaty food, salt, sugar, condiments, fried, and preserved foods; tobacco, flesh meat, and liquor also should be avoided.

Hay fever :—treat like Fever.

Haemorrhage:—bleeding from any orifice of the body—cold water compress covered with flannel bandage; in bleeding from the nose, put it over the nose and the region of the liver also. Non-stimulating diet.

Haemorroids or piles:—Avoid heaty food which is likely to cause constipation; keep a cold compress over the region of the liver covered with flannel bandage. In obstinate cases use massage over the region of the liver and expose the part to the sun.

Heatstroke:—Pour tepid water over the head and neck and massage the parts very slowly and gently so that the blood may be carried to the region of the heart and the lower parts of the body. Give only fruit juice to the patient till he feels better; later on give hot foot-bath with cold compress over the head once or twice daily till the patient feels all right and keep him on non-stimulating diet.

Hernia:—Hahn recommends for the cure of hernia 5 to 6 weeks' perfect rest in bed; natural diet *i. e* milk and fruits; avoidance of all sorts of exertion; daily four to five washings of the abdomen;—daily massage in the form of friction with circular movements around the place of rupture and four times a day the application of stimulating abdominal fomentation with stimulating thick extra compresses on the site of the rupture. If all this is carefully done Hahn asserts that the truss is then a superfluity (Platen).

Hoarseness:—Shower bath, sunbath or massage to the throat and the region of larynx.

Hydrophobia:—Steam-bath followed by Hip-bath and Sun-bath or brisk walks; avoid all food not meant by Nature for human consumption, chiefly sugar, salt, pickles and fried things at least for a year after the bite.

Hydrothorax or Dropsy of the chest:—Sun-bath daily or steam bath on alternate days followed by hip-bath and brisk walk; diet—milk and fruit juice only, avoid salt, sugar and salted-food.

Hypochondriasis—Morbid anxiety about one's own health:—shower bath on head, neck and spine followed by sun-bath; non-stimulating diet, occasional fasting for 24 hours. In most obstinate cases hip-bath followed by a brisk walk.

Hysteria:—See Nervous diseases.

Impotence and sexual weakness are the resu[illegible] of sexual wrongs previously committed; they may be caused on account of sexual excess, disease of the testicles or spinal cord or a bad type of dyspepsia. They may also be caused by venereal diseases, fright, worry, grief, over-exertion of the mind, too long an abstinence, over indulgence in tobacco, liquor, cocaine, etc. or the frequent use of contraceptive remedies:—Hip-bath twice a day of 72° temperature followed by sun bath; Massage on spine; suitable exercise.—See chapter IX; non-stimulating diet, milk, fruits and nuts are chiefly recommended. Avoid all exciting causes and stimulating drinks and the use of narcotics, spices, etc. Try to obey Nature in every respect.

Impotence:—(1) Mr. G. of S. was completely impotent. All the remedies tried had availed nothing. By means of my treatment which he carried out at home consisting of alternate friction, sitz and hip-baths and a non-flesh diet his disorder was perfectly cured within six weeks (Kuhne).

(2) A strong and fat man aged 32 was impotent. Ayurvedic, Unani, Allopathic and patent remedies were not able to produce the desired effect; steam baths weekly, hip-baths and sunbaths daily with morning and evening walks and natural diet made him all right in three months (Author).

Inflammation :—All inflammatory conditions, such as Appendicitis, Arthritis, Balanitis, Bronchitis, Cystitis, Enteritis simple or tubercular, Gastritis, Iritis, Laryngitis, Meningitis, Metritis, Nephritis, Orchitis, Otitis, Pericarditis, Peritonitis, Pleuritis, Pneumonia, Phlebitis, Rhinitis, Tonsillitis, etc. are to be treated with cold water bandage, sunbath, fasting, diet, breathing exercise, enema, and massage.

Influenza :—see cold and catarrhal fever.

Insanity :—Douche-bath on head as long as possible for several days till the patient gets healthy sleep at night or till he catches severe cold. As a rule, insanes do not catch cold, nor do they get sound sleep. Shower bath over the head, neck and spine followed by sunbath.

In obstinate cases avoid all narcotics, stimulating drinks, spices, liquors and flesh-meat. Give only milk and fruits; also keep a watch over the patient and see whether he is addicted to any sexual wrongs; if so do not allow him to commit them. If he does not get sleep give him hot footbath also and keep him on salt and sugar-free diet. See Nervous diseases also.

Insomnia, sleeplessness :—Avoid coffee, tea and all stimulating drinks, narcotics, flesh-meat and hot drinks; give hot footbath every night and make him take long walks in bright sunlight and keep his bowels moved daily by the use of an enema.

Iritis—see Diseases of eyes.

Jaundice, as a rule is caused on account of liver disorders :—Avoid oily and fatty food, keep bowels clear by the aid of an enema. Massage or sunbath over the region of the liver, non-stimulating diet and walking exercise.

Liver, Cirrhosis of, (interstitial inflammation) :—Sunbath, cold water compress, massage, and enema; light, easily digestible food well masticated and insalivated before swallowing. Congestion of liver :—cold water compress and massage or sun-bath.

Lumbago, Neuralgia of the loins:—very hot fomentation, tepid enema and massage over the affected part. In obstinate cases steam-bath and hip-bath; avoid flesh-meat, pulses and wind producing substances.

Lupus, Tuberculosis of the skin appearing on the face :—steam-bath and hipbath; sunbath on the affected part after washing it with soapnut-water. Vegetable diet, non-stimulating food; tobacco, liquor, coffee, and aerated waters should be avoided. The author has cured four obstinate cases of lupus with the aforesaid treatment and Homeopathic medicines.

Lupus :—" My system of treatment produced very successful results in the case of a lady in *Stettin*. The patient had suffered from *lupus* of the face for 19 years and she could no longer show her face to any one. She always wore a thick veil in order to conceal her disfigured face. All the remedies at the command of medical science had been tried unsuccessfully for 19 years by this lady before she came to me; under my treatment, improvement at once began and a cure was soon effected" (Kuhne)

Masturbation or self abuse is the worst of all offences against Nature. The perpetrator may turn sexually weak or impotent and may suffer from any nervous disease, e.g. epilepsy, paralysis, insomnia, or insanity, see chapter IV; keep a strict watch over the person suspected of this offence and advise him not to commit it explaining the consequences of it:—Non-stimulating diet, sunbath followed by hip-bath and brisk walk and control over the mind may save the patient from the worst results. Many young persons have been saved from its ill-effects by proper advice and useful hints to avoid the habit. They afterwards left the habit and became successful both as students and citizens.

Nervous diseases:—All nervous disorders such as nervous debility, neuralgia, neuritis, nervousness, sleeplessness, convulsions, chorea, hysteria, neurasthenia, hypochondriasis, epilepsy, infantile paralysis, locomotor ataxia, palsy, insanity, cramps, in any part of the body, spasmodic troubles of all kinds are to be treated with hipbath, sunbath, enema, fruit diet, hot foot bath and shower bath.

The author has cured several cases of convulsions, hysteria, neuritis, nervousness, sleeplessness, chorea, epilepsy, paralysis, insanity, etc. with the above treatment. In some obstinate cases however he had to make use of mesmerism, hypnotism, suggestions and homeopathic medicines also.

"It may confidently be asserted that many nervous disorders are really caused by the employment of drugs which have at first been administered to cure some less serious complaints. As for the cure of nervous diseases, it cannot be denied that the much lauded medical profession stands utterly helpless. Indeed its representatives have frequently confessed their total inability to aid in such cases (Kuhne).

St. Vitus' dance and Sleeplessness :—

"Daugther of Mrs. G. of L. was afflicted with these troubles. Her whole body being in convulsions ; she was neither able to walk nor speak, she was unable to sleep, hold any thing or to digest her food. After having tried all manner of cures the patient came under my treatment. Hip and friction sitz baths, the latter much prolonged, exercise in fresh air and suitable diet soon had the desired effect" (Kuhne).

"**Nervous spasms** (fits)—Mrs. G. suffering from peculiar spasms. These commenced in the finger tips and passed to the head causing the patient the greatest trouble. The most eminent physicians of the place had treated the patient but without any success, on the contrary she became much worse. Friction sitz baths and natural diet improved her and she was all right in seven weeks" (Kuhne).

Insanity :—" A girl of 23 who had been afflicted for several years with total insanity was brought to me by her parents to whom she was a constant source of anxiety. The condition of the patient was such that she could not even bathe herself, her mother having to do it for her. In four weeks however she was so far improved that she could take the baths herself and was no longer uncleanly in her habits; within half a year she could again be reckoned among the healthy members of the family" (Kuhne).

Obesity :—sugar free and starch free diet, avoidance of oily and fatty-food and fried things; cold friction baths early morning and brisk walks in the bright sunlight have cured several persons of their corpulence in most obstinate cases; Phytolacca berry preparations have proved very efficacious. If the patient is too fat and over-anxious to reduce his fat, give him steambaths followed by hipbaths and brisk walks.

Paralysis :—sunbath, shower-bath and massage. Non-stimulating diet; avoid spices, tobacco, liquor, coffee, tea, wines and fleshmeat; use an enema to keep the bowels clean; the patients will improve steadily and have a complete cure. See also nervous diseases.

Poisonous bites—Rat bites, mad dog bites, mad jackal bites, etc. :—Steam-baths, hipbaths and sun-baths; salt free diet. Avoid fried things and keep bowels moved daily by the use of an enema.

Snake bite:—A young woman of 20 was bitten in the foot by a snake; her foot and leg began to swell and she suffered great agony. Physicians declared that she cannot be cured. She had lost consciousness and she was more dead than alive. Then her father made a last desperate effort to save her by resorting to a remedy which tradition said had saved a girl bitten by a snake centuries ago. He dug a hole in the garden put his daughter naked into it and then covered her up leaving only her head free. The girl was dug up again after twenty four hours later completely cured (Just).

Poisons:—Anacardium poisoning (poison from marking nut tree), ivy poisoning (poison from rhus tree), gout, lumbago, rheumatism, (acute or chronic), gonorrhoeal or syphilitic uremia, septicæmia, toxemia, etc. should be treated with sun-bath and cold water bandage; diet and enema are also necessary. In obstinate cases try steam and hipbaths.

Opium, arsenic and other poisons swallowed wilfully or by mistake :—make the patient vomit by tickling in the throat with a feather and making the patient drink ample tepid water; empty the colon with an enema. Give also sun-bath and make the patient drink water exposed to sunlight in a Blue bottle.

Poisonous effects of serums, vaccines and other injections and ill effects of vaccination are to be treated with sunbath daily, and steam bath twice a week.

Polypus is a smooth pedunculated growth from a mucous surface. See Scientific Hydropathy for the treatment.

Prostate is a gland surrounding the neck of the bladder and the end of urethra like a ring. In young or old persons grey hair indicates its affection; the enlargement of it can be cured by massage treatment; see chapter X. Sabal Serrulata, Natrum sulph, Ferrum phos, Thuja, Lycopodium are the homeopathic remedies which effect wonderful cures in prostatic troubles.

Respiratory organs:—Bronchitis, croup, diphtheria, coughs of all sorts, colds, influenza, hay fever, laryngitis, pharyngitis, pleurisy, pneumonia, whooping cough, etc. are to be treated with sunbaths and hipbaths. Frequent air baths and occasional sponge baths are also necessary. If bowels are constipated an enema should be tried occasionally. All oily and fatty substances should be avoided; milk and fruits in season are recommended.

The chief causes of lung disease are the wearing of too tight clothing, inhaling of foul air and chiefly the air mixed with vapour coming on while frying foodstuffs, smoke, anti-septic remedies, powerful scents, strong odoured drugs, etc. In restaurants those who are engaged on frying duty as a rule die of pneumonia or phthisis pulmonalis; so also Phthisis pulmonalis and pneumonia are more common among women who are engaged in cooking and frying than among men who attend outdoor work and are not required to do such work. By excess of clothing and tight wearing of dress the skin is smothered and is not allowed to help lungs in inhaling oxygen which is a mighty blood purifier and powerful eliminator of carbonic acid and waste matter from the organism.

Rheumatism:—Treat like an inflammatory disease. See Scientific Hydropathy and Practical Chromopathy by the author.

Rickets :—Rub the whole body with cocoanut juice and give sun-bath daily; milk, fruit juice, and oatmeal conjee recommended. Wheat conjee may be given. See Practical Chromopathy and Scientific Hydropathy by the author.

Skin-diseases :—Acne, barber's itch, dandruff, eruptions, herpes, hives, impetigo, scurf, eczema of all kinds, itches, scabies, vesicles, pruritus, prurigo, eruptions of all kinds, and all other skin diseases are the result of impure blood. Keep the bowels regular by the use of an enema; light, natural, non-stimulating diet; use pure cold water and soap-nut water during bathing and to wash the affected parts. In obstinate cases steambath once a week and hip-bath daily. Do not use bazaar soap.

Several most obstinate skin complaints have been cured by the author with the above treatment and homœopathic remedies; the patients insisted to have some medicines both internally and externally.

A *sore* or ulcer or even the most obstinate eczema, may be cured by applying external remedies. But as these are the result and outcome of internal impurities of the blood and as they are the natural efforts of the great healer Nature, to drive out or expel such impurities through the skin, the purulent matter if forced back in the blood will do greater harm to the body. It will cause more impurities by coming in contact with the healthy tissue and causing more mortification or rotten condition in flesh and blood. Pyorrhœa is not the disease of the teeth nor of the gum but an unhealthy condition of the blood and Nature finds an easy outlet from the orifices of the gums to expel the morbid matter. By removing the teeth discharge of pus may no doubt be stopped but it will cause more harmful effect in the flesh and blood unless the blood is purified by natural diet, air and sun baths, external and internal water baths, proper exercise and by desisting from those habits which have caused that condition, such as smoking or eating tobacco, drinking hot and strong tea, coffee, ærated waters, liquors, etc. and also eating sweetmeats, spiced foods, fried things, etc. There are instances of persons having suffered from other serious troubles in such cases when the teeth were removed and the discharge stopped in an unnatural way.

Snake bite :—the author had no occasion to try natural methods alone in such cases. He did not get a single case of cobra bite as yet for the treatment. He had several occasions to treat the bites of carpet snakes and other venomous snakes. Homeopathic remedies were tried as the patients and their relatives desired the Homeopathic medical treatment in addition to the steambath recommended; the patients were recommended salt free diet for some days.

Spermatorrhoea—Night emissions, sexual weakness and impotency are as a rule the results of sexual sins, such as, masturbation, onanism, the use of French letters and pessaries as contraceptive remedies, sexual starvation or sexual excess, long continued use of opium, cocaine or tobacco, drinking habits, etc. They cause stimulation first and later on the total weakness or complete inability amounting to impotency. As such ailments are caused by disobeying Nature, the best way to cure such troubles is to obey her only; natural intercourse with a woman whom you love and who loves you in return will cure the trouble. Sitz bath, shower bath, hipbath, sunbath, fruit diet and enema are the auxiliary remedies needed.

Sycosis and spinal neuralgia:—Mr. H. had been for years suffering from sycosis. All the parts about the beard had become deep red and was covered with scales and tubercles. The patient had tried all the possible treatment without success. Several friction baths daily, suitable diet and two steam-baths weekly cured him in 5 months. (Kuhne)

Syphilis:—See Scientific Hydropathy. Two patients agreed to take sun-bath directly on the affected part through green glass in addition to the other treatment and they got cured sooner than the patients otherwise treated. Microbes disappear when the blood is purified.

Syphilis:—Baron V. E. aged 47 Consulted me some years ago for syphilis for which he had four times undergone the Allopathic treatment by mercurial *injection* at the hands of eminent doctors. He had likewise been dosed with *potassium iodide*; but in spite of all this the syphilitic symptoms always returned and open sores in the mouth and on the feet made their appearance. As a consequence he lost all faith in Allopathy, the more so as his general health after the mercurial treatment was no longer nearly so good as formerly. More recently he had suffered from a feeling of oppression in the head and he had lost his clear memory. It was quite clear that syphilis had been rendered latent by the Mercurial treatment. Steambaths, hip-baths and natural diet cured him entirely in 6 months (Kuhne).

Tetanus, continuous tonic spasm of muscle:—Fomentations, massage and sunbath. In obstinate cases neutral bath. Diet--milk and friuts only; enema to keep the bowels clear.

Tonsillitis, inflammation of the tonsils:—It can be cured without operation; massage and sunbath; throat pack (see Scientific Hydropathy); non-stimulating diet.

Tooth-ache :—Foment. In obstinate cases foment the parts with heated sand, massage and sunbath are also very useful.

Tuberculosis :—See consumption for Tuberculosis of lungs (phthisis) and bowels (Tabes mesenterica); for tuberculosis of bones, lymph-glands (scrofula) if unsuppurated try massage and sunbath or local steambath, and cold friction; if suppurated sunbath and fomentation with hot sand; fruits and milk diet, wholemeal wheat or maize bread; fleshmeat, spices, tobacco and liquor forbidden. For tuberculosis of skin see Lupus.

Tumours :—Massage and sunbath. In obstinate cases, local steambath and cold compress covered with flannel. Avoid flesh-meat, condiments and narcotics.

Ulcer :—Treat like skin diseases.

Uremia :—Steam-bath and hip-bath ; non-stimulating diet ; enema for constipation. An ounce of water prepared according to chromopathic principles in a green bottle twice a day morning and bedtime.

Vaccination, ill effects of :—steam-bath and hip-bath, cold water friction bath in the morning followed by a brisk walk in the sun.

Varicocele, dilatation and elongation of the veins and spermatic cords :—Local steam bath ; massages with cold water. In obstinate cases hip bath also and enema in case of constipation.

Varicose veins :—try like varicocele ; massage will greatly help.

Whooping cough :—Massage to chest and long neutral bath. In obstinate cases hip-bath and sun bath.

Worms :—Full enema of soap-nut water ; soap nut water compress over the region of navel. In obstinate cases hip-bath and water medicated in blue bottle by keeping it in the sun according to chromopathic principles. Lemon juice diluted in water or milk with a little honey but not sugar, under-ripe, acid or sub-acid fruits and wholemeal bread. Avoid fleshmeat, sugar preparations and over-eating.

Writer's cramp :—Massage and shower bath and sun-bath also when available.

Wry neck :—Treat like rheumatism. Massage, shower-bath and sun-bath are very necessary, avoid stimulating and wind producing food; avoid flesh meat and pulses; keep bowels clean and take proper exercise.

Zymotic diseases :—eruptive fevers such as small-pox, chicken-pox, measles, German measles, scarlet fever, erysipelas, etc. are to be treated with breathing exercise, water compress, enema, and diet.

FINIS

ERRATA.

Page.	Line	For	Read.
1	14	संगं	संगो
1	14	कारकम्	कारकः
2	6	निश्रेयसायन:	निःश्रेयसे तव
37	15	breath	breathe
38	8	mak	make
55	3	Statagem	stratagem
67	12 omit 4 lines from "Are in the blood .... found in it."		
89	19	expectration	expectoration
132	5	Shool	School
138	7	Vigonr	Vigour
141	27	digestve	digestive
236	1	exelaimed	exclaimed
238	18	premitive	primitive

Plate I

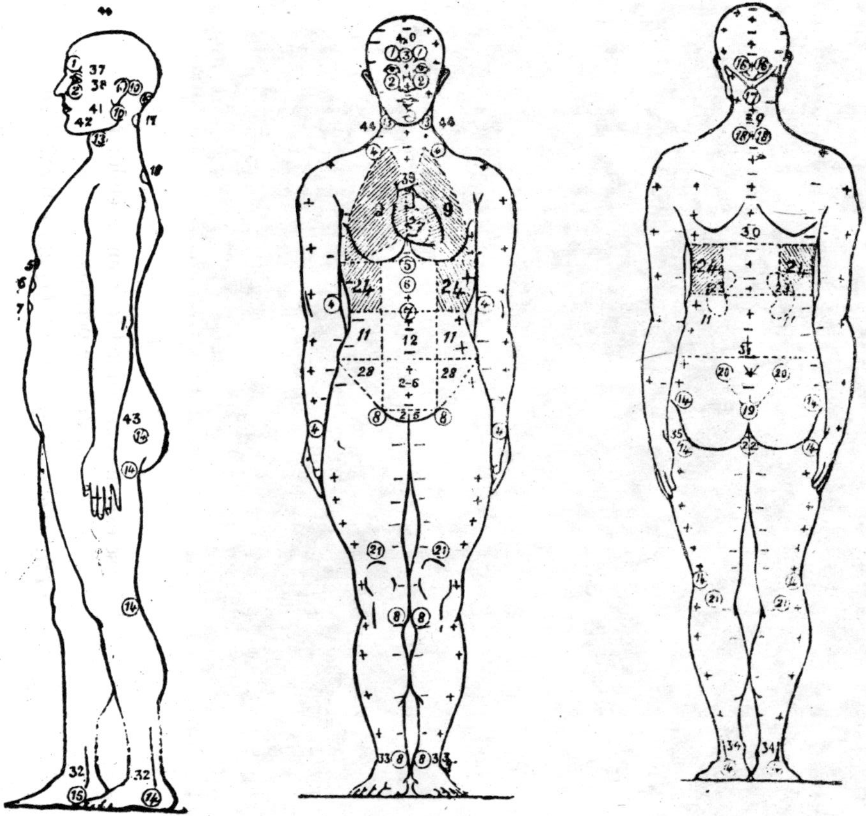

\+ Plus is positive

− Minus is negative

5 Solar Plexus

6 Pit of Stomach

7 Gastric Sympathetic

9 Lungs

14 Sciatic Nerve

17 Occipital Nerves

18 Crural Sympathetic

23 Kidneys

24 Hypochondria

27 Heart

See Page 168

Plate II

2

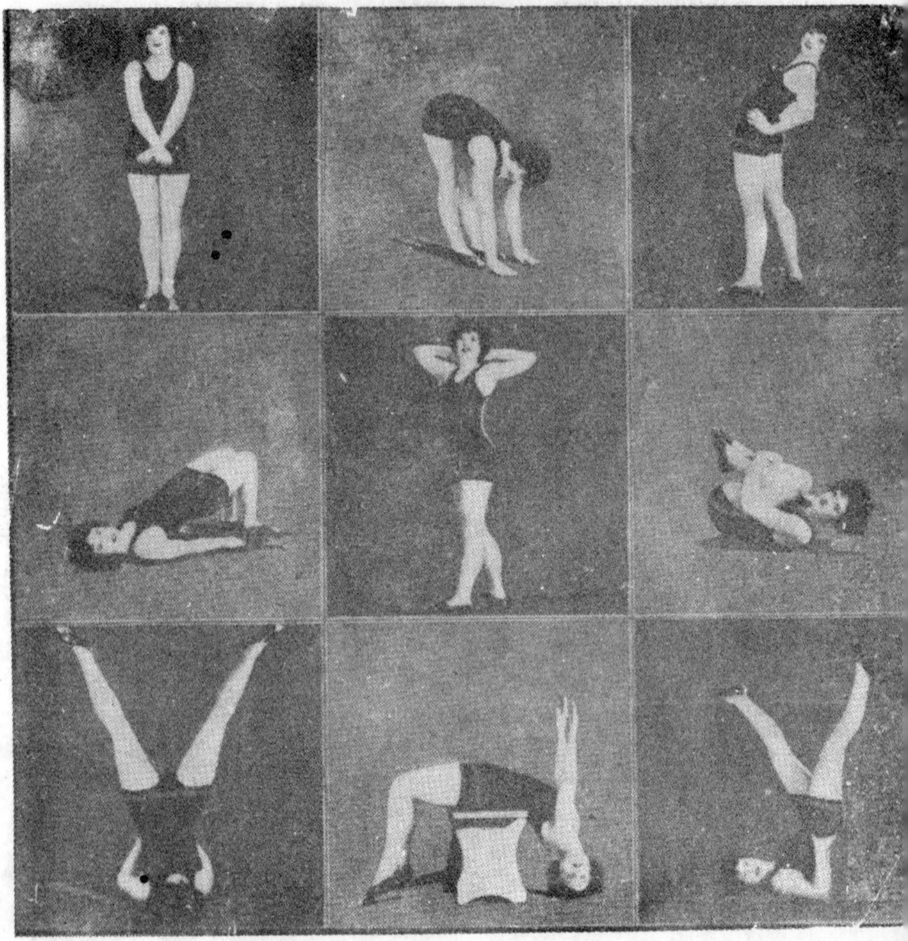

8

These exercises are suited to women, children and delicate persons.

From Physicial Culture with apologies to Macfadden.

Plate III

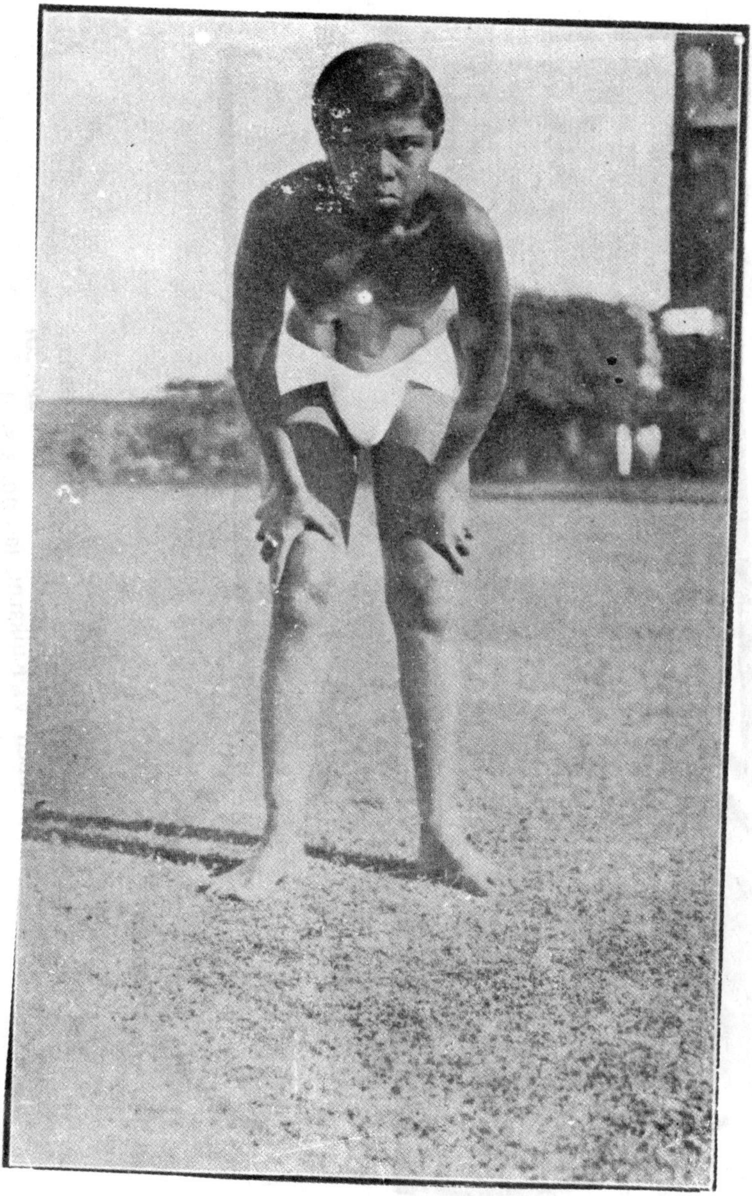

Nauli by Ratnakar V. Kulkarni, (author's son)
Ex. 21, Page 204

Plate IV

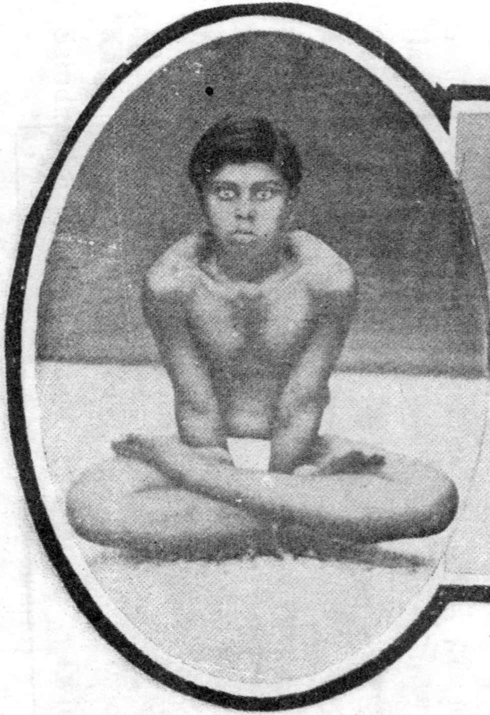

Yogasana
Ex. 22, Page 204

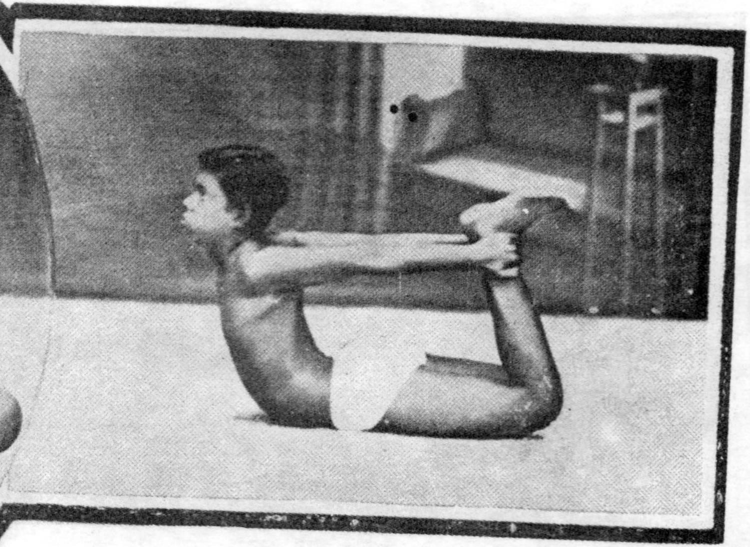

Dhanurasana
Ex. 28, Page 207

By Ratnakar V. Kulkarni, (author's son)

Plate V

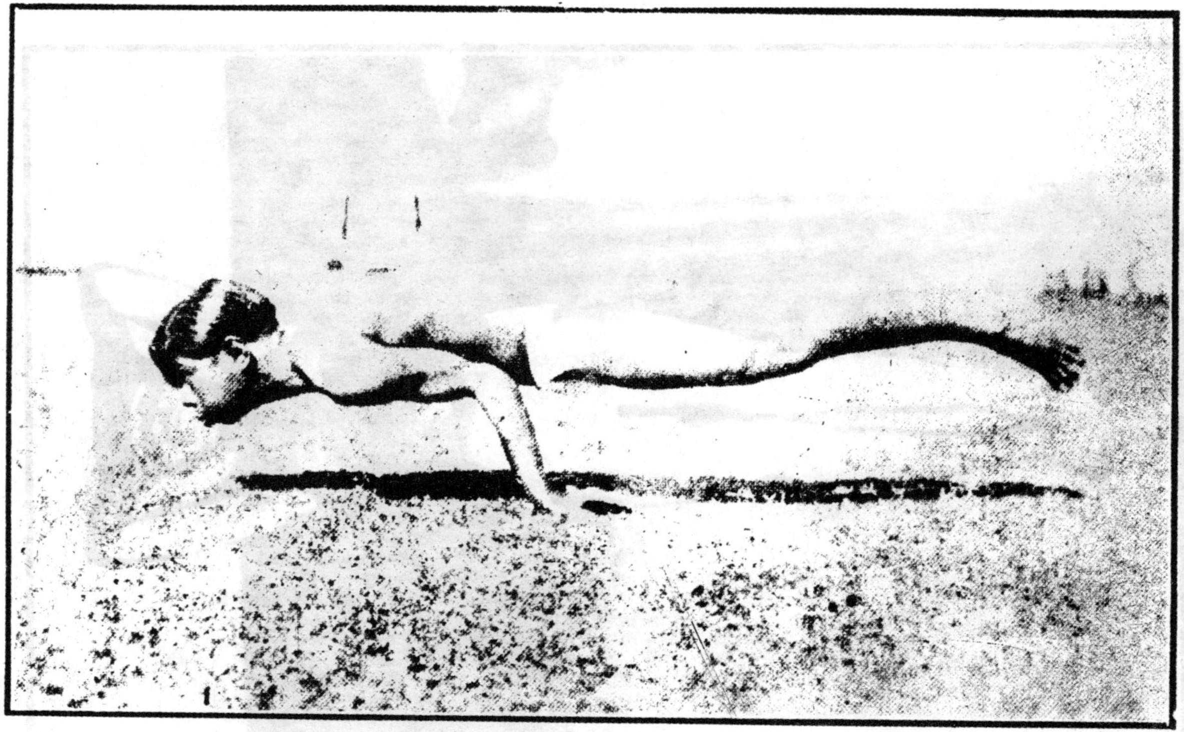

Mayurasana by Ratankar V. Kulkarni

Ex. 26, Page 206

Plate VI

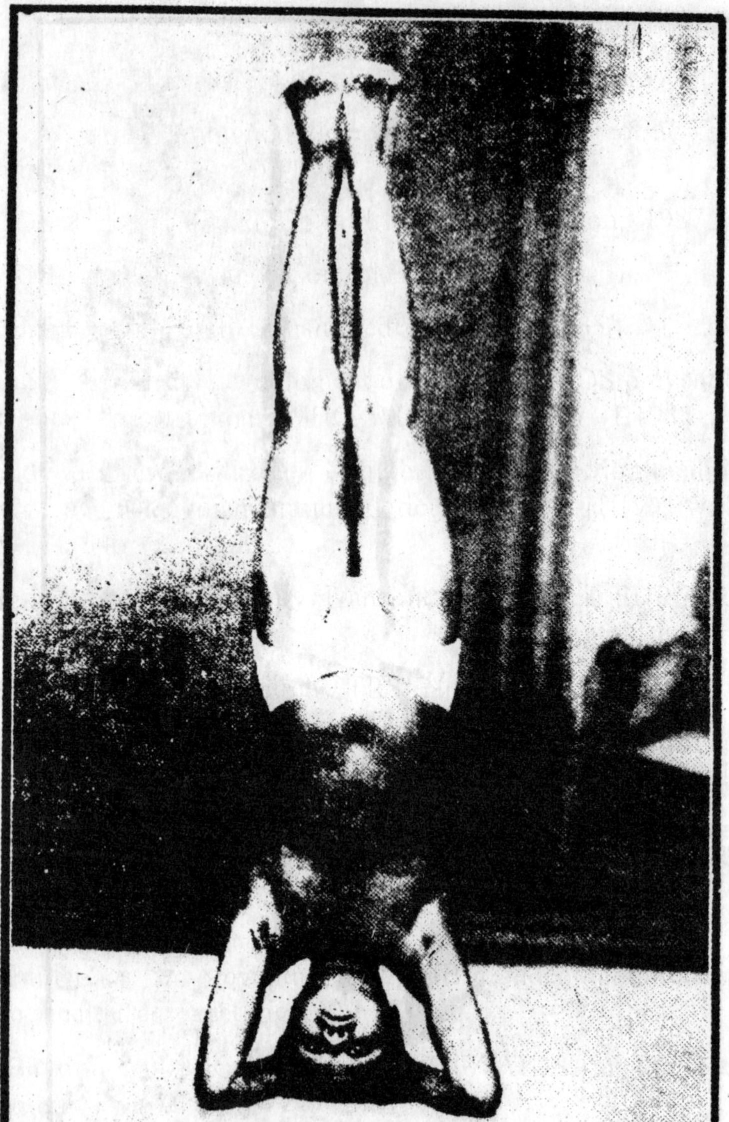

Shirshasana by Ratnakar V. Kulkarni, (author's son)
Ex. 31, Page 209

Plate VII

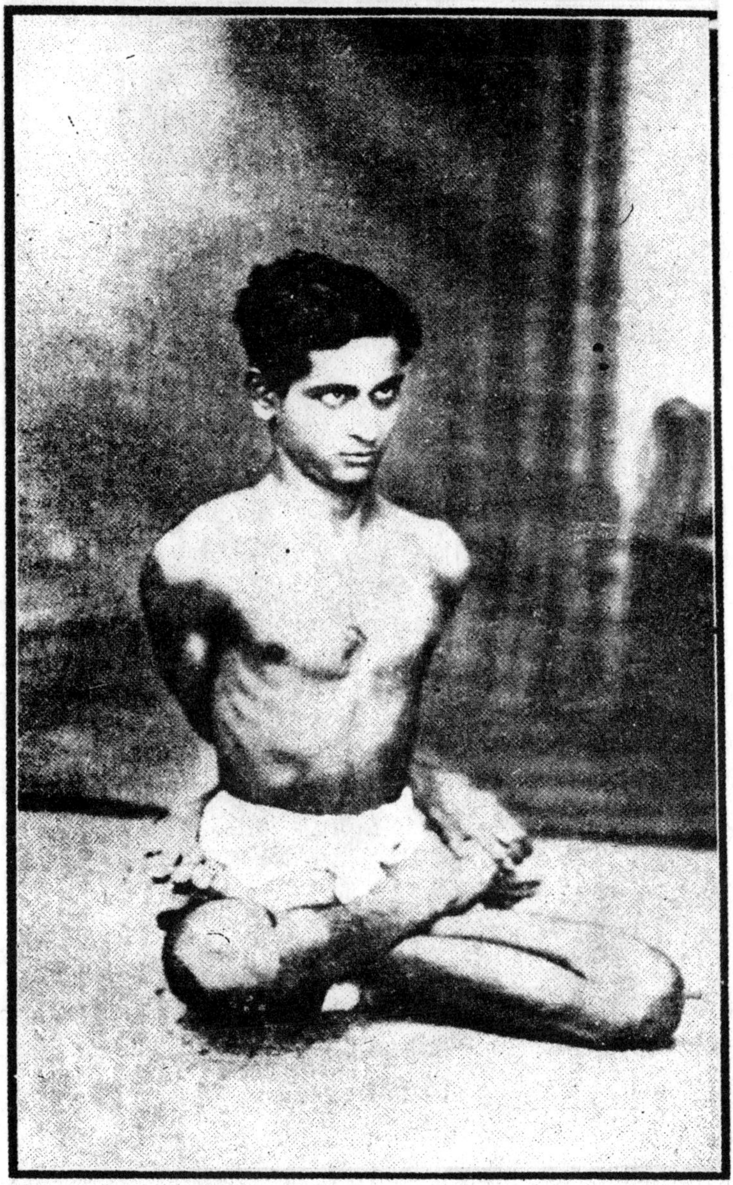

Padmasana by G. N. Kulkarni, (author's nephew)
Ex. 24, Page 205

Plate VIII

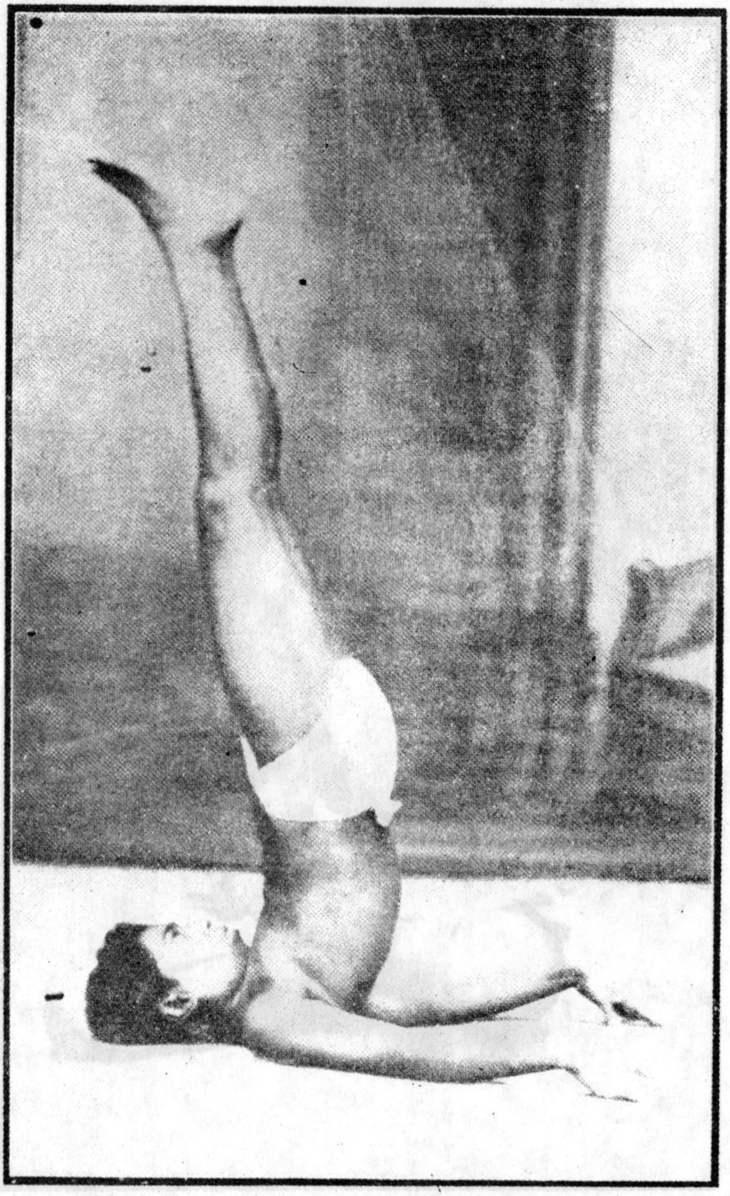

Sarwangasana by Ratnakar V. Kulkarni. (author's son)
Ex. 32, Page 210

Plate IX

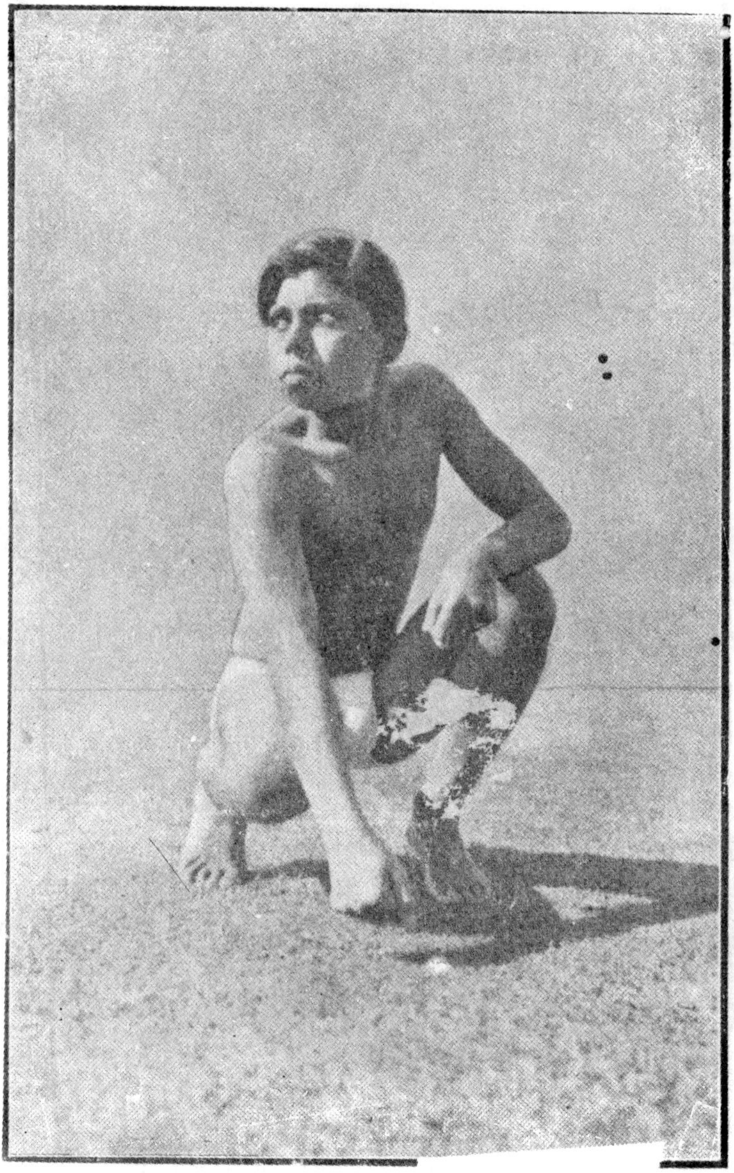

Ratnakar V. Kulkarni
Ex. 20, Page 201

Plate X

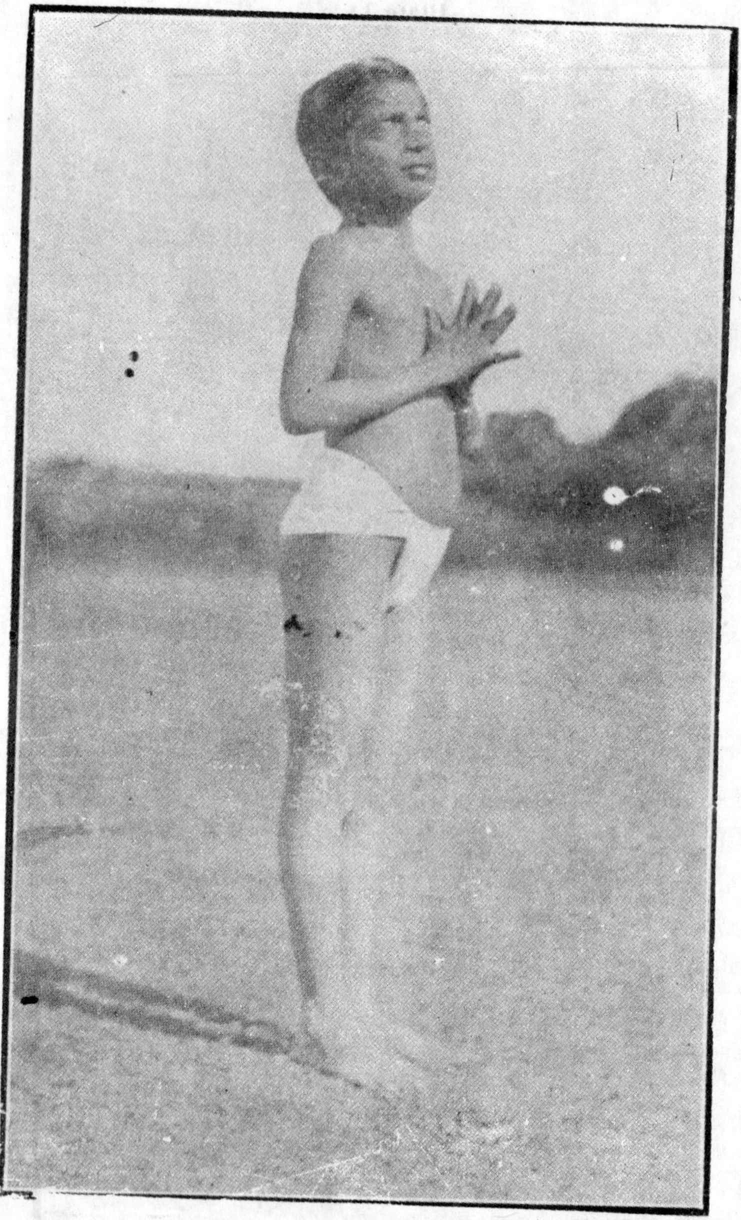

Soorya Namaskar by Ramesh R. Kulkarni, (author's grandson)

Page 189